Mosby's
PHYSICAL
EXAMINATION
HANDBOOK

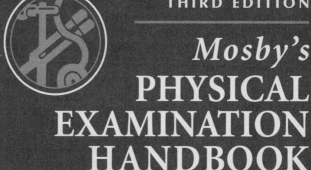

THIRD EDITION

Mosby's PHYSICAL EXAMINATION HANDBOOK

HENRY M. SEIDEL, MD
Professor Emeritus of Pediatrics
The Johns Hopkins University School of Medicine
Baltimore, Maryland

JANE W. BALL, RN, DRPH, CPNP
Executive Director
National Resource Center
Children's National Medical Center
Washington, DC

JOYCE E. DAINS, DRPH, JD, RN, CS, FNP
Assistant Professor
Department of Family and Community Medicine
Baylor College of Medicine
Houston, Texas

G. WILLIAM BENEDICT, MD, PHD
Assistant Professor, Medicine
The Johns Hopkins University School of Medicine
Baltimore, Maryland

Mosby

An Affiliate of Elsevier Science

St. Louis   London   Philadelphia   Sydney   Toronto

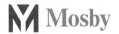

An Affiliate of Elsevier Science

11830 Westline Industrial Drive
St. Louis, MO 63146

Notice

Health care is an ever-changing field. Standard safety precautions must be followed, but as new research and clinical experience broaden our knowledge, changes in treatment and drug therapy may become necessary or appropriate. Readers are advised to check the most current product information provided by the manufacturer of each drug to be administered to verify the recommended dose, the method and duration of administration, and contraindications. It is the responsibility of the licensed prescriber, relying on experience and knowledge of the patient, to determine dosages and the best treatment for each individual patient. Neither the publisher nor the editor assumes any liability for any injury and/or damage to persons or property arising from this publication.

The Publisher

Previous editions copyrighted 1995, 1999.

Library of Congress Cataloging-in-Publication Data

Mosby's physical examination handbook / Henry M. Seidel . . . [et al.].—3rd ed.
    p. ; cm
  Includes bibliographical references and index.
  ISBN 0-323-01679-0
   1. Physical diagnosis—Handbooks, manuals, etc. I. Title: Physical examination handbook. II. Seidel, Henry M.
   [DNLM: 1. Physical Examination—methods—Handbooks. WB 39 M894 2003]
RC76 .M64 2003
616.07'54—dc21

2002019266

Vice President and Publishing Director: Sally Schrefer
Managing Editor: Lee Henderson
Publishing Services Manager: Deborah L. Vogel
Project Manager: Deon Lee
Design Manager: Bill Drone

GW/QWT

Printed in the United States of America.

Last digit is the print number: 9 8 7 6 5 4 3 2 1

Preface

Mosby's Physical Examination Handbook, third edition, is a portable clinical reference on physical examination suitable for students of nursing, medicine, chiropractic, and other allied health disciplines, as well as for practicing health care providers. It offers brief descriptions of examination techniques and guidelines on how the examination should proceed, step by step. This handbook is intended to be an aid to review and recall of the procedures of physical examination. It cannot, because of its brevity, describe the specific techniques of history taking by organ system.

The handbook begins with an outline of what information should be obtained for the patient's medical history and review of systems. Subsequent chapters for each of the body systems list equipment needed to perform the examination and present the techniques to be used. Expected and unexpected findings follow the description of each technique, presented in distinctive color type for easy recognition. Numerous illustrations interspersed throughout the text reinforce techniques and possible findings.

Each chapter offers Aids to Differential Diagnosis and also provides Sample Documentation, which in this edition has been focused on a specific complaint to illustrate good documentation practice. Pediatric Variations are also highlighted in each body systems chapter.

As in previous editions, separate chapters give an overview of the entire examination for all adults; for healthy females; and for infants, children, and adolescents. The final chapter gives guidelines for reporting and recording findings.

New to this edition is the separation of the Heart and Blood Vessels chapter into two chapters: Heart (10) and Blood Vessels (11). This change should make examination of each system more efficient.

Also new to this edition is an appendix of special histories. This appendix includes the CAGE questionnaire (for detecting alcoholism), the TACE questionnaire (for detecting risk drinking), the RAFFT questionnaire (for detecting substance abuse in adolescents), and several additional special histories.

The summary card found at the back of this book is included for your convenience. It is intended as a quick pocket reference to supplement both the handbook and *Mosby's Guide to Physical Examination*, fifth edition.

Henry M. Seidel
Jane W. Ball
Joyce E. Dains
G. William Benedict

Contents

MERLIN mosby.com/MERLIN/Seidel

The History

TAKING THE HISTORY

The following outline of what to include when taking a patient history should be viewed not as a rigid structure but as a general guideline. Since you are beginning your relationship with the patient at this point, pay attention to this relationship as well as to the information you seek in the history. Be friendly and show respect for the patient. Choose a comfortable setting and help the patient get settled. Maintain eye contact and use a conversational tone. Begin by introducing yourself and explaining your role. Help the patient understand why you are taking the history and how it will be used. Once the history proceeds, explore positive responses with additional questions: Where, when, what, how, and why. Be sensitive to the patient's emotions at all times. Avoid confrontation and asking leading questions.

CHIEF COMPLAINT

Problem or symptom: Reason for visit
Duration of problem
Patient information: Age, sex, marital status, previous hospital admissions; occupation
Other complaints: Secondary issues, fears, concerns, what made patient seek care

PRESENT PROBLEM

Chronologic ordering: Sequence of events patient has experienced
State of health just before onset of present problem
Complete description of first symptom: Time and date of onset, location, movement

Possible exposure to infection or toxic agents

If symptoms are intermittent, describe typical attack: Onset, duration, symptoms, variations, inciting factors, exacerbating factors, relieving factors

Impact of illness: On lifestyle, on ability to function; limitations imposed by illness

"Stability" of problem: Intensity, variations, improvement, worsening, staying same

Immediate reason for seeking attention, particularly for long-standing problem

Review of appropriate system when there is a conspicuous disturbance of a particular organ or system

Medications: Current and recent, dosage of prescriptions, home remedies, nonprescription medications

Review of chronology of events for each problem: Patient's confirmations and corrections

MEDICAL HISTORY

General health and strength

Childhood illnesses: Measles, mumps, whooping cough, chickenpox, smallpox, scarlet fever, acute rheumatic fever, diphtheria, poliomyelitis

Major adult illnesses: Tuberculosis (TB), hepatitis, diabetes, hypertension, myocardial infarction, tropical or parasitic diseases, other infections, any nonsurgical hospital admissions

Immunizations: Poliomyelitis, diphtheria, pertussis, tetanus toxoid, influenza, *Haemophilus influenzae* B, pneumococcal, cholera, typhus, typhoid, bacille Calmette-Guérin (BCG), hepatitis B virus (HBV), last purified protein derivative (PPD) or other skin tests; unusual reactions to immunizations; tetanus or other antitoxin made with horse serum

Surgery: Dates, hospital, diagnosis, complications

Serious injuries: Resulting disability (document fully for injuries with possible legal implications)

Limitation of ability to function as desired as a result of past events

Medications: Past, current, recent medications; dosage of prescription; home remedies and nonprescription medications, particularly complementary and alternative therapies

Allergies: Especially to medications but also to environmental allergens and foods

Transfusions: Reactions, date, number of units transfused

Emotional status: Mood disorders, psychiatric treatment
Children: Birth, developmental milestones, childhood diseases, immunizations

FAMILY HISTORY

Relatives with similar illness
Immediate family: Ethnicity, health, cause of and age at death
History of disease: Heart disease, high blood pressure, hypercholesterolemia, cancer, TB, stroke, epilepsy, diabetes, gout, kidney disease, thyroid disease, asthma and other allergic states, forms of arthritis, blood diseases, sexually transmitted diseases, other familial diseases
Spouse and children: Age, health
Hereditary disease: History of grandparents, aunts, uncles, siblings, cousins; consanguinity

PERSONAL AND SOCIAL HISTORY

Personal status: Birthplace, where raised, home environment; parental divorce or separation, socioeconomic class, cultural background, education, position in family, marital status, general life satisfaction, hobbies and interests, sources of stress and strain
Habits: Nutrition and diet; regularity and patterns of eating and sleeping; exercise: quantity and type; quantity of coffee, tea, tobacco, alcohol; illicit drug use: frequency, type, amount; breast or testicular self-examination
Sexual history: Concerns with sexual feelings and performance, frequency of intercourse, ability to achieve orgasm, number and gender of partners
Home conditions: Housing, economic condition, type of health insurance if any, pets and their health
Occupation: Description of usual work and present work if different; list of job changes; work conditions and hours; physical and mental strain; duration of employment; present and past exposure to heat and cold, industrial toxins (especially lead, arsenic, chromium, asbestos, beryllium, poisonous gases, benzene, and polyvinyl chloride or other carcinogens and teratogens); any protective devices required, for example, goggles or masks
Environment: Travel and other exposure to contagious diseases, residence in tropics, water and milk supply, other sources of infection if applicable

Military record: Dates and geographic area of assignments

Complementary and alternative health and medical systems: History and current use

Religious preference: Religious proscriptions concerning medical care

Cost of care: Resources available to patient, financial worries, candid discussion of issues

REVIEW OF SYSTEMS

General constitutional symptoms: Fever, chills, malaise, fatigability, night sweats, weight (average, preferred, present, change)

Diet: Appetite, likes and dislikes, restrictions (because of religion, allergy, or disease), vitamins and other supplements, use of caffeine-containing beverages (coffee, tea, cola), an hour-by-hour detailing of food and liquid intake—sometimes a written diary covering several days of intake may be necessary

Skin, hair, nails: Rash or eruption, itching, pigmentation or texture change, excessive sweating, abnormal nail or hair growth

Musculoskeletal: Joint stiffness, pain, restriction of motion, swelling, redness, heat, bony deformity

Head and neck:

General: Frequent or unusual headaches, their location, dizziness, syncope, severe head injuries, periods of loss of consciousness (momentary or prolonged)

Eyes: Visual acuity, blurring, diplopia, photophobia, pain, recent change in appearance or vision, glaucoma, use of eye drops or other eye medications, history of trauma or familial eye disease

Ears: Hearing loss, pain, discharge, tinnitus, vertigo

Nose: Sense of smell, frequency of colds, obstruction, epistaxis, postnasal discharge, sinus pain

Throat and mouth: Hoarseness or change in voice, frequent sore throats, bleeding or swelling of gums, recent tooth abscesses or extractions, soreness of tongue or buccal mucosa, ulcers, disturbance of taste

Endocrine thyroid enlargement or tenderness, heat or cold intolerance, unexplained weight change, diabetes, polydipsia, polyuria, changes in facial or body hair, increased hat and glove size, skin striae

Males: Puberty onset, erections, emissions, testicular pain, libido, infertility

Females:

Menses: Onset, regularity, duration and amount of flow, dysmenorrhea, date of last period, intermenstrual discharge or bleeding, itching, date of last Pap smear, age at menopause, libido, frequency of intercourse, sexual difficulties, infertility

Pregnancies: Number, miscarriages, abortions, duration of pregnancy, type of delivery for each, any complications during any pregnancy or postpartum period or with neonate, use of oral or other contraceptives

Breasts: Pain, tenderness, discharge, lumps, galactorrhea, mammograms (screening or diagnostic), frequency of breast self-examination

Chest and lungs: Pain related to respiration, dyspnea, cyanosis, wheezing, cough, sputum (character and quantity), hemoptysis, night sweats, exposure to TB, date and result of last chest x-ray examination

Heart and blood vessels: Chest pain or distress, precipitating causes, timing and duration, character, relieving factors, palpitations, dyspnea, orthopnea (number of pillows needed), edema, claudication, hypertension, previous myocardial infarction, estimate of exercise tolerance, past electrocardiogram (ECG) or other cardiac tests

Hematologic: Anemia, tendency to bruise or bleed easily, thromboses, thrombophlebitis, any known abnormality of blood cells, transfusions

Lymph nodes: Enlargement, tenderness, suppuration

Gastrointestinal: Appetite, digestion, intolerance of any class of foods, dysphagia, heartburn, nausea, vomiting, hematemesis; regularity of bowels, constipation, diarrhea, change in stool color or contents (clay colored, tarry, fresh blood, mucus, undigested food), flatulence, hemorrhoids; hepatitis, jaundice, dark urine; history of ulcer, gallstones, polyps, tumor; previous x-ray examinations (where, when, findings)

Genitourinary: Dysuria, flank or suprapubic pain, urgency, frequency, nocturia, hematuria, polyuria, hesitancy, dribbling, loss in force of stream, passage of stone, edema of face, stress incontinence, hernias, sexually transmitted disease (inquire type and symptoms and results of serologic test for syphilis, if known)

Neurologic: Syncope, seizures, weakness or paralysis, abnormalities of sensation or coordination, tremors, loss of memory

Psychiatric: Depression, mood changes, difficulty concentrating, nervousness, tension, suicidal thoughts, irritability, sleep disturbances

PEDIATRIC VARIATIONS

Taking the history

These are only guidelines; you are free to modify and add as the needs of your patients and your judgment dictate.

Chief complaint

A parent or other responsible adult will generally be the major resource. However, when age permits, child should be involved as much as possible. Remember that every chief complaint has the potential of an underlying concern. What really led to the visit to you? Was it just the sore throat?

Reliability

Note relationship to patient of person who is the resource for history, and record your impression of the competence of that person as a historian.

Present problem

Be sure to give a clear chronologic sequence to the story.

Medical history

In general, the age of the patient and/or the nature of the problem will guide your approach to the history. Clearly, in a continuing relationship much of what is to be known will already have been recorded. Certainly, different aspects of the history require varying emphasis depending on the nature of the immediate problem. There are specifics that will command attention.

 Pregnancy/mother's health:
    Infectious disease; give approximate gestational month
    Weight gain/edema
    Hypertension
    Proteinuria
    Bleeding; approximate time
    Eclampsia, threat of eclampsia
    Special or unusual diet or dietary practices
    Medications (hormones, vitamins)
    Quality of fetal movements, time of onset
    Radiation exposure
    Prenatal care/consistency
 Birth and perinatal experience:
    Duration of pregnancy

Delivery site

Labor: Spontaneous/induced, duration, anesthesia, complications

Delivery: Presentation; forceps/spontaneous; complications

Condition at birth: Time of onset of cry; Apgar scores, if available

Birth weight and, if available, length and head circumference

Neonatal period:

Hospital experience: Length of stay, feeding experience, oxygen needs, vigor, color (jaundice, cyanosis), cry. Did baby go home with mother?

First month of life: Color (jaundice), feeding, vigor, any suggestion of illness or untoward event

Feeding:

Bottle or breast: Any changes and why; type of formula, amounts offered/taken, feeding frequency; weight gain

Present diet and appetite: Introduction of solids, current routine and frequency, age weaned from bottle or breast, daily intake of milk, food preferences, ability to feed self; elaborate on any feeding problems

Development

Guidelines suggested in Chapter 21, Age-Specific Examination: Infants, Children, and Adolescents, are complementary to the milestones listed below. Those included here are commonly used, often remembered, and often recorded in "baby books." Photographs may also be of some help occasionally.

Age when:

Held head erect while held in sitting position

Sat alone, unsupported

Walked alone

Talked in sentences

Toilet trained

School: Grade, performance, learning and social problems

Dentition: Ages for first teeth, loss of deciduous teeth, first permanent teeth

Growth: Height and weight at different ages, changes in rate of growth or weight gain or loss

Sexual: Present status (e.g., in female, time of breast development, nipples, pubic hair, description of menses; in males, development of pubic hair, voice change, acne, emissions). Follow Tanner guides.

Family history

Maternal gestational history: All pregnancies with status of each, including date, age, cause of death of all deceased siblings and dates and duration of pregnancy in the case of miscarriages; mother's health during pregnancy

Age of parents at birth of patient

Are parents related to each other in any way?

Personal and social history

Personal status:
    School adjustment
    Nail biting
    Thumb sucking
    Breath holding
    Temper tantrums
    Pica
    Tics
    Rituals
Home conditions:
    Parental occupation(s)
    Principal caretaker(s) of patient
    Food preparation, routine, family preferences (e.g., vegetarianism), who does preparing
    Adequacy of clothing
    Dependency on relief or social agencies
    Number of persons and rooms in house or apartment
    Sleeping routines and sleep arrangements for child

Review of systems (some suggested additional questions or particular concerns)

Ears: Otitis media (frequency, laterality)
Nose: Snoring, mouth breathing
Teeth: Dental care
Genitourinary: Nature of urinary stream, forceful or a dribble
Skin, hair, nails: Eczema or seborrhea

2

Mental Status

EQUIPMENT

- Familiar objects (coins, keys, paper clips)
- Paper and pencil

EXAMINATION

Perform the mental status examination throughout the patient inter-action. Focus on the individual's strengths and capabilities for execu-tive functioning (motivation, initiative, goal formation, planning and performing work or activities, self-monitoring, and integrating feed-back from various sources to refine or redirect energy). Interview a family member or friend if you have any concerns about the patient's responses or behaviors.

Use a mental status screening examination for health visits when no cognitive, emotional, or behavior problems are apparent. Information is generally observed during the history in the follow-ing areas:

Appearance and behavior
   Grooming
   Emotional status
   Body language

Cognitive abilities
   State of consciousness
   Memory
   Attention span
   Judgment

Emotional stability
   Mood and feelings
   Thought process and content

Speech and language
   Voice quality
   Articulation
   Comprehension
   Coherence
   Ability to communicate

TECHNIQUE	FINDINGS

Mental Status and Speech Patterns

Observe physical appearance and behavior

- *Grooming*

  UNEXPECTED: Poor hygiene; lack of concern with appearance; or inappropriate dress for season, gender, or occasion in previously well-groomed patient.

- *Emotional status*

  EXPECTED: Patient expressing concern with visit that is appropriate for emotional content of topics discussed.

  UNEXPECTED: Behavior conveying carelessness, indifference, inability to sense emotions in others, loss of sympathetic reactions, unusual docility, rage reactions, agitation, or excessive irritability.

- *Body language*

  EXPECTED: Erect posture and eye contact (if culturally appropriate).

  UNEXPECTED: Slumped posture, lack of facial expression, inappropriate affect, excessively energetic movements, or constantly watchful eyes.

Investigate cognitive abilities

- *Six-Item Cognitive Impairment Test*
  Use this test to assess cognition (see p. 11).

  EXPECTED: Score less than 10.
  UNEXPECTED: Score between 10 and 28.

- *Mini-Mental State Examination (MMSE)*
  Use this examination to quantify cognitive function or document changes.

  EXPECTED: Score of 21-30.
  UNEXPECTED: Score of 20 or less.

Six-Item Cognitive Impairment Test

Item	Maximum Error	Score	Weight	Final Item Score
1. What *year* is it now?	1		4	
2. What *month* is it now?	1		3	
Memory phrase: Repeat this phrase after me: *"John Brown, 42 Market Street, Chicago"*				
3. About what time is it now? (within an hour)	1		3	
4. Count backwards 20 to 1	2		2	
5. Say the months in reverse order	2		2	
6. Repeat the memory phrase	5		2	

Assign 0 for a correct score, and 1 for each incorrect score up to the maximum number of errors permitted. Multiply the item score by the item weight to obtain the final item score. The maximum total score possible is 28. A score of 10 or higher is significant and should be referred.

From Brooke, Bullock, 1999.

TECHNIQUE	FINDINGS
MMSE can be obtained from the following: Psychological Assessment Resources, Inc PO Box 998 Odessa, FL 33556 Phone: 1-800-331-8378	
■ *State of consciousness*	**EXPECTED:** Oriented to time, place, and person, and able to appropriately respond to questions and environmental stimuli. **UNEXPECTED:** Disoriented to time, place, or person. Verbal response is confused, incoherent, or inappropriate, or there is no verbal response.
■ *Set Test* Use this test to evaluate mental status as a whole (motiva-	**EXPECTED:** Able to categorize, count, remember items listed. Score of 25 or more points.

TECHNIQUE	FINDINGS

tion, alertness, concentration, short-term memory, problem solving). Ask patient to name 10 items in each of 4 groups: fruit, animals, colors, town/cities. Give each item 1 point for a maximum of 40 points.

UNEXPECTED: Score less than 15 points. Check for mental changes or cultural, educational, or social factors when score is 15 to 24.

■ *Analogies*
Ask patient to describe analogies, first simple, then more complex:
  ▪ What is similar about peaches and lemons, oceans and lakes, pencil and typewriter?
  ▪ An engine is to an airplane as an oar is to a _____?
  ▪ What is different about a magazine and a telephone book, or a bush and a tree?

UNEXPECTED: Unable to describe similarities or differences.

■ *Abstract reasoning*
Ask patient to explain meaning of fable, proverb, or metaphor:
  ▪ A stitch in time saves nine.
  ▪ A bird in the hand is worth two in the bush.
  ▪ A rolling stone gathers no moss.

UNEXPECTED: Unable to give adequate explanation.

■ *Arithmetic calculations*
Ask patient to perform simple calculations without paper and pencil:

UNEXPECTED: Unable to complete with few errors within a minute.

TECHNIQUE	FINDINGS

- 50 − 7, − 7, − 7, etc., until answer is 8.
- 50 + 8, + 8, + 8, etc., until answer is 98.

■ *Writing ability*
Ask patient to write name and address or a phrase you dictate (or draw simple figures—triangle, circle, square, flower, house— if unable to write).

UNEXPECTED: Omission or addition of letters, syllables, or words; mirror writing; or uncoordinated writing (or drawing for patients unable to write).

■ *Execution of motor skills*
Ask patient to do a motor task such as combing hair.

UNEXPECTED: Unable to complete a task.

■ *Memory*
Immediate recall: Ask patient to listen to, then repeat, a sentence or series of numbers (five to eight numbers forward, four to six numbers backward).
Recent memory: Show patient four or five objects or give visually impaired patient four unrelated words with distinct sounds to remember (carpet, iris, bench, fortune). Say you will ask about them later. In 10 minutes, ask patient to list objects.
Remote memory: Ask patient about verifiable past events (e.g., mother's maiden name, name of high school).

EXPECTED: *Immediate recall:* Able to repeat sentence or numbers.
Recent memory: Able to remember test objects.
Remote memory: Able to recall verifiable past events.
UNEXPECTED: Impaired memory. Loss of immediate and recent memory with retention of remote memory.

■ *Attention span*
Ask patient to follow a series of short commands (e.g., take off all clothes, put on patient gown, sit on examining table).

EXPECTED: Responds to directions appropriately.
UNEXPECTED: Easy distraction or confusion, negativism.

TECHNIQUE	FINDINGS

■ *Judgment*
Explore:
  ▪ How patient meets social and family obligations, patient's future plans.
  ▪ Patient's solutions to hypothetical situations (e.g., found stamped envelope or was stopped for running red light).
	EXPECTED: Able to evaluate situation and provide appropriate response; managing business affairs appropriately.
	UNEXPECTED: Response indicating hazardous behavior or inappropriate action

Evaluate emotional stability

■ *Mood and feelings* Ask patient how he or she feels, whether feelings are a problem in daily life, and whether he or she has particularly difficult times or experiences.	**EXPECTED:** Appropriate feelings for the situation. **UNEXPECTED:** Unresponsiveness, hopelessness, agitation, euphoria, irritability, or wide mood swings.
■ *Geriatric Depression Scale* Use this test to assess for possible depression in older adults (see p. 15).	**EXPECTED:** Score of 5 or less. **UNEXPECTED:** Score greater than 5.

■ *Thought process and content*
  ▪ Ask patient about obsessive thoughts and compulsive behaviors.
  ▪ Observe sequence, logic, coherence, and relevance of topics.
	EXPECTED: Patient's thought processes can be followed, and expressed ideas are logical and goal directed.
	UNEXPECTED: Illogical or unrealistic thought process, blocking, or disturbance in stream of thinking. Obsessive thought content or behavior that interferes with daily life or is disabling.

■ *Perceptual distortions and hallucinations* Ask patient about any sensations not believed caused by external stimuli. Find out when these experiences occur.	**UNEXPECTED:** Auditory, visual, or tactile hallucinations—hears voices, sees vivid images or shadowy figures, smells offensive odors, feels worms crawling on skin.

Geriatric Depression Scale (short form)
Ask the patient to choose the best answer for how he felt over the previous week.

1. Are you basically satisfied with your life?	YES / NO
2. Have you dropped many of your activities and interests?	YES / NO
3. Do you feel that your life is empty?	YES / NO
4. Do you often get bored?	YES / NO
5. Are you in good spirits most of the time?	YES / NO
6. Are you afraid that something bad is going to happen to you?	YES / NO
7. Do you feel happy most of the time?	YES / NO
8. Do you feel helpless?	YES / NO
9. Do you prefer to stay at home, rather than going out and doing new things?	YES / NO
10. Do you feel you have more problems with memory than most?	YES / NO
11. Do you think it is wonderful to be alive now?	YES / NO
12. Do you feel pretty worthless the way you are now?	YES / NO
13. Do you feel full of energy?	YES / NO
14. Do you feel that your situation is hopeless?	YES / NO
15. Do you think most people are better off than you are?	YES / NO

Correct responses are the following:
  Yes for questions 2, 3, 4, 6, 8, 9, 10, 12, 14, and 15.
  No for questions 1, 5, 7, 11, and 13.
Give one point for each correct answer. A score greater than five suggests depression.

From Sheikh, Yesavage, 1986.

TECHNIQUE	FINDINGS
Observe speech and language	
■ *Voice quality*	**EXPECTED:** Uses inflections, speaks clearly and strongly, is able to increase voice volume and pitch. **UNEXPECTED:** Difficulty or discomfort making laryngeal speech sounds or varying volume, quality, or pitch of speech.
■ *Articulation*	**EXPECTED:** Proper pronunciation, fluent, rhythmic; easily expresses thoughts. **UNEXPECTED:** Imperfect pronunciation, difficulty articulating single speech sound, rapid-fire delivery, or speech with hesitancy, stuttering, repetitions, or slow utterances.

TECHNIQUE	FINDINGS
■ *Comprehension*	**EXPECTED:** Able to follow simple instructions.
■ *Coherence*	**EXPECTED:** Able to clearly convey intentions or perceptions.
	UNEXPECTED: Circumlocutions, perseveration, flight of ideas or loosening of associations between thoughts, gibberish, neologisms, clang association, echolalia, or unusual sounds.
■ *Ability to communicate*	**UNEXPECTED:** Hesitations, omissions, inappropriate word substitutions, circumlocutions, neologisms, disturbance of rhythm or words in sequence or other signs of aphasia.

AIDS TO DIFFERENTIAL DIAGNOSIS

ABNORMALITY	DESCRIPTION
Dementia	Insidious onset; depressed, apathetic mood persists. Rambling or incoherent speech. Memory, judgment, thought patterns, calculations impaired. Progressive condition.
Delirium	Sudden onset; condition lasts for hours or days. Mood and affect include rapid mood swings, fear, suspicion. Slurred or rapid and manic speech and hallucinations are common. Sleep-wake cycle may be disturbed.

ABNORMALITY	DESCRIPTION
Dementia of Alzheimer's type	Subtle, insidious onset—generally with early memory loss, impaired ability to learn new information, or disturbance in executive functioning—leading to profound disintegration of personality and complete disorientation. Varied duration and rate of progression.
Depression	Altered mood and affect with extreme sadness, anxiety, irritability. Lack of motivation, lethargic or restless and agitated. Poor concentration.
Anxiety disorder	Marked anxiety or fear that interferes with personal, social, occupational functioning. Panic attacks with symptoms such as palpitations, tachycardia, sweating, shaking, trembling, choking, chest pain, abdominal distress, dizziness, faintness.
Mental retardation	Subaverage intellectual functioning, deficits in adaptive behavior, inability to discriminate among stimuli, impaired short-term memory, lack of motivation.

PEDIATRIC VARIATION
EXAMINATION

TECHNIQUE	FINDINGS

Mental Status

Use parent's impressions of infant's responsiveness to guide your assessment	**EXPECTED:** Infant responds appropriately to parent's voice—is attentive, comforts easily. Child follows simple directions, performs age-appropriate skills (Chapter 21).

AIDS TO DIFFERENTIAL DIAGNOSIS

ABNORMALITY	DESCRIPTION
	UNEXPECTED: Nonresponsive, inconsolable, combative, lethargic.
Autistic disorder	Development disorder with odd repetitive behaviors, preoccupation with objects, an aversion to touch, delayed language or echolalia. Motor development may progress as expected.
Attention-deficit hyperactivity disorder	Developmentally inappropriate inattention, hyperactivity, impulsivity, temper bursts, labile moods.

SAMPLE DOCUMENTATION

Subjective. A 16-year-old male fell playing basketball and struck the back of his head on a wooden floor. No loss of consciousness, got up and walked immediately, was dazed and confused for a few moments, has a headache.

Objective. Oriented to time, place, person. Reasoning and arithmetic calculation abilities intact. Immediate, recent, and remote memory intact. Appropriate mood and feeling expressed. Speech clearly and smoothly enunciated. Comprehends directions.

3

Nutrition and Growth and Measurement

EQUIPMENT

- Tape measure with millimeter markings
- Calculator
- Skinfold caliper

EXAMINATION

TECHNIQUE	FINDINGS

Anthropometrics

Measure height and weight

- *Estimate desirable body weight (DBW).*
Add 10% for large frame; subtract 10% for small frame.

EXPECTED: *Women:* 100 pounds for first 5 feet; plus 5 pounds for each inch thereafter. *Men:* 106 pounds for first 5 feet; plus 6 pounds for each inch thereafter.

- *Use growth charts for pediatric patients (pp. 292-299).*

EXPECTED: Child is following a growth curve pattern for height and weight. Height and weight are approximately same percentiles.

- *Calculate % weight change*

$$\left(\frac{\text{Usual weight} - \text{Current weight}}{\text{Usual weight}} \right) \times 100$$

UNEXPECTED: Weight loss that equals or exceeds 1% to 2% in 1 week, 5% in 1 month, 7.5% in 3 months, 10% in 6 months.

TECHNIQUE	FINDINGS
■ *Calculate body mass index (BMI) (kg/m²)*	**EXPECTED:** 18.5 to 24.9 for both men and women.

$$\left(\frac{\text{Weight in pounds} \times 703}{\text{Height in inches}} \right) \div$$

Height in inches
or see nomogram below.

EXPECTED: 18.5 to 24.9 for both men and women.
UNEXPECTED: BMI above 30.0 corresponds with obesity class I.

Nomogram for body mass index (kg/m²). Weight/height² is read from the central scale. The ranges suggested as "desirable" are from life insurance data.

From Thomas AE et al, 1976.

TECHNIQUE   FINDINGS

Calculate waist-to-hip circumference ratio

Using tape measure with millimeter markings, measure waist
at or 1 cm above umbilical midline. Then measure hip at level
of superior iliac crest. Divide
waist circumference by hip circumference to obtain the ratio.

EXPECTED: Ratio less than 0.9
in men and 0.8 in women.
UNEXPECTED: Ratios over 0.9
in men and 0.8 in women indicate increased central fat distribution and increased risk of
disease.

Midarm muscle circumference (MAMC)

■ *Measure mid upper arm circumference (MAC)*

Place tape around upper right
arm, midway between tips of olecranon and acromial processes.
Hold tape snugly and make the
reading to nearest 5 mm.
This measurement is obtained
to calculate midarm muscle circumference (MAMC).

EXPECTED: Between 10th and
95th percentiles.
UNEXPECTED: Less than 10th
or greater than 95th percentile
(see table below).

Percentiles for Midarm Circumference, Midarm Muscle Circumference, and Triceps Skinfold

	Men		Women	
Percentile	55-65 years	65-75 years	55-65 years	65-75 years
Arm Circumference (MAC), cm				
10th	27.3	26.3	25.7	25.2
50th	31.7	30.7	30.3	29.9
95th	36.9	35.5	38.5	37.3
Arm Muscle Circumference (MAMC), cm				
10th	24.5	23.5	19.6	19.5
50th	27.8	26.8	22.5	22.5
95th	32.0	30.6	28.0	27.9
Triceps Skinfold (TSF), mm				
10th	6	6	16	14
50th	11	11	25	24
95th	22	22	38	36

From Frisancho AR, 1981.

TECHNIQUE	FINDINGS

■ *Measure triceps skinfold (TSF) thickness*

Have patient flex right arm at a right angle. Find midpoint between tips of olecranon and acromial process, and make a horizontal mark. Then draw a vertical line to intersect. With arm relaxed, use your thumb and forefinger to grasp and lift triceps skinfold about ½ inch proximal to intersection marks. Place caliper at skinfold and measure without making an indentation. Make two readings to nearest millimeter, and derive an average.

This measurement is obtained to calculate MAMC.

EXPECTED: Between 10th and 95th percentiles.

UNEXPECTED: Less than 10th or greater than 95th percentile (see table on p. 21).

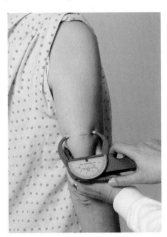

■ *Calculate MAMC*

MAMC = {MAC (mm) − [3.14 × TSF (mm)]}

Compare measurement to table for percentiles.

EXPECTED: Between 10th and 95th percentiles.

UNEXPECTED: Less than 10th or greater than 95th percentile (see table on p. 21).

Calculate estimates for energy needs

Use actual weight for healthy adults
Use adjusted weight for obese patients

Adjusted weight = [(Actual body weight − DBW) × 25%] + DBW

CALORIES	KCAL/KG
Weight loss	25
Weight maintenance	30
Weight gain	35
Hypermetabolic/ malnourished	35-50

TECHNIQUE	FINDINGS

Biochemical Measurements

Obtain biochemical measures as indicated

Hemoglobin	**EXPECTED:** See reference ranges established by your particular laboratory.
Hematocrit	
Serum albumin	
Transferrin saturation	
Serum glucose	
Triglycerides	
Cholesterol	
High-density lipoprotein (HDL) cholesterol	
Low-density lipoprotein (LDL) cholesterol	
Serum folate	

AIDS TO DIFFERENTIAL DIAGNOSIS

ABNORMALITY	DESCRIPTION
Obesity	Exogenous obesity characterized by excess fat located in breast, buttocks, thighs. Associated with excessive caloric intake, thick skin, pale striae, preservation of muscle strength, no evidence of osteoporosis. Endogenous obesity characterized by excess fat tissue distributed to certain regions of the body such as trunk or abdominal areas.
Anorexia nervosa	Psychologic disorder in which person has a relentless drive for thinness through self-imposed starvation, bizarre food habits, obsessive exercise, self-induced vomiting or laxative abuse. Condition characterized by weight loss to 85% or less of expected weight or failure to attain expected weight. Common signs and symptoms include those of starvation.

Comparison of Laboratory Test Results for Anemias

Test	Normal Value	Iron Deficiency Anemia	Folic Acid Deficiency Anemia	Vitamin B$_{12}$ Deficiency Anemia
Hemoglobin, 100 g/ml	Men: 14-16 Women: 12-14	Decreased	Decreased	Decreased
Hematocrit, %	Men: 40-54 Women: 37-47	Decreased	Decreased	Decreased
Mean corpuscular volume (MCV), μm³	82-92	Decreased (<80)	Increased (>92)	Increased (>92)
Mean corpuscular hemoglobin (MCH), pg	27-31	Decreased (<27)	Increased (>35)	Increased (>35)
Mean corpuscular hemoglobin concentration (MCHC), %	32-36	Decreased (<32)	Normal	Normal
Serum iron, μg/100 ml	60-180	Decreased	Increased	Increased
Total iron-binding capacity (TIBC), μg/100 ml	250-450	Increased (>350)	Normal	Normal
Transferrin saturation, %	20-55	Decreased (<20)	Normal	Normal

ABNORMALITY	DESCRIPTION
Bulimia	Eating disorder characterized by binge eating, followed by self-induced vomiting. Patient usually does not become malnourished unless body weight continues to drop to less than 85% of expected weight.
Anemias	Lowering of serum hemoglobin and hematocrit levels and change in size, appearance, and production of red blood cells; common symptoms include pallor, weakness, fatigue, headache, dizziness (see table on p. 24).
Hyperlipidemia	High blood cholesterol (240 g/100 ml) defined as value above which risk for coronary heart disease sharply rises (see box below and table on p. 26).

Major Risk Factors That Modify Low-Density Lipoprotein Goals*†

- Cigarette smoking
- Hypertension (blood pressure ≥140/90 mm Hg or use of antihypertensive medication)
- Low high-density lipoprotein cholesterol (<40 mg/100 ml)‡
- Family history of premature coronary heart disease (in male first-degree relative <55 years; in female first-degree relative < 65 years)
- Age (men ≥45 years; women ≥55 years)

From National Cholesterol Education Program Expert Panel on Detection, Evaluation, and Treatment of High Blood Cholesterol in Adults (Adult Treatment Panel III), 2001.
*Exclusive of low-density lipoprotein cholesterol.
†In Adult Treatment Panel III, diabetes is regarded as a coronary heart disease risk equivalent.
‡HDL cholesterol ≥60 mg/100 ml counts as a "negative" risk factor; its presence removes one risk factor from the total count.

Three Categories of Risk That Modify Low-Density Lipoprotein Cholesterol Goals

Risk Category	LDL Goal (mg/100 ml)
Coronary heart disease (CHD) and CHD risk equivalents	<100
Multiple (+2) risk factors	<130
0 or 1 risk factor	<160

From National Cholesterol Education Program Expert Panel on Detection, Evaluation, and Treatment of High Blood Cholesterol in Adults (Adult Treatment Panel III), 2001.

PEDIATRIC VARIATIONS
EXAMINATION

TECHNIQUE	FINDINGS
Measure head circumference	
Wrap tape measure snugly around infant's head at occipital protuberance and supraorbital prominence.	Refer to growth charts for infants and children.
Calculate estimates for energy needs	
Pediatric patients: 1000 kcal plus 100 kcal per year of age, up to age 12 years. *Fat:* Over age 2 years, less than 30% of daily calories from fat; before age 2 years, fat intake of 35% to 40% of calories.	

SAMPLE DOCUMENTATION

Subjective. A 45-year-old business man with steady weight gain over the past 5 years. Seeks nutrition counseling for weight loss plan. Eats three full meals each day with snacking in between; eats breakfast and dinner at home, where wife prepares meals. Often eats lunch (fast foods) on the run. Alcohol intake: 1 to 2 glasses of wine daily with dinner. No regular exercise. Has never kept a meal log. No change in lifestyle; moderate stress.

Objective. Height: 173 cm (68 inches). Weight: 90.9 kg (200 pounds), 123% of desirable body weight; BMI: 30.5; triceps skinfold thickness: 20 mm, 90th percentile; midarm circumference: 327.8 mm; midarm muscle circumference: 265 mm, 25th percentile; 2200 calories daily estimated for appropriate weight loss.

4

Skin, Hair, and Nails

EQUIPMENT

- Centimeter ruler (flexible, clear)
- Flashlight with transilluminator
- Wood's lamp
- Magnifying glass (optional)

EXAMINATION

TECHNIQUE	FINDINGS
Skin	
Perform overall inspection of entire body	
In particular, check areas not usually exposed and intertriginous surfaces.	**EXPECTED:** Skin color differences among body areas and between sun-exposed and non–sun-exposed areas. **UNEXPECTED:** Lesions.

TECHNIQUE   FINDINGS

Inspect skin of each body area and mucous membranes

- *Color/uniformity*
  Inspect sclerae, conjunctivae, buccal mucosa, tongue, lips, nail beds, and palms of dark-skinned patients for color hues.

EXPECTED: General uniformity—dark brown to light tan, with pink or yellow overtones. Sun-darkened areas. Darker skin around knees and elbows. Callused areas yellow. Knuckles darker and palms/soles lighter in dark-skinned patients. Vascular-flush areas pink or red, especially with anxiety or excitement. Pigmented nevi. Nonpigmented striae. Freckles. Birthmarks.

Purpura—red-purple nonblanch-able discoloration greater than 0.5 cm diameter.
Cause: Intravascular defects, infection

Petechiae—red-purple nonblanch-able discoloration less than 0.5 cm diameter
Cause: Intravas-cular defects, infection

Ecchymoses—red-purple non-blanchable discoloration of variable size
Cause: Vascular wall destruction, trauma, vasculitis

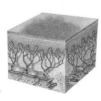

Spider angioma—red central body with radiating spi-derlike legs that blanch with pressure to the central body
Cause: Liver disease, vitamin B deficiency, idiopathic

Venous star—bluish spider, linear or irregularly shaped; does not blanch with pressure
Cause: Increased pressure in superficial veins

Telangiectasia—fine, irregular red line
Cause: Dilation of capillaries

Capillary hemangioma (nevus flammeus)—red irregular macular patches
Cause: Dilation of dermal capillaries

TECHNIQUE	FINDINGS
	UNEXPECTED: Dysplastic, pre-cancerous, or cancerous nevi. Chloasma. Unpigmented skin. Generalized or localized color changes. Vascular skin lesions. Vascular changes.

Cutaneous Color Changes

Color	Cause	Distribution	Select Conditions
Brown	Darkening of melanin pigment	Generalized	Pituitary, adrenal, liver disease
		Localized	Nevi, neuro-fibromatosis
White	Absence of melanin	Generalized	Albinism
		Localized	Vitiligo
Red (erythema)	Increased cutaneous blood flow	Localized	Inflammation
		Generalized	Fever, viral exan-thems, urticaria
	Increased intra-vascular red blood cells	Generalized	Polycythemia
Yellow	Increased bile pigmentation (jaundice)	Generalized	Liver disease
	Increased carotene pig-mentation	Generalized (except sclera)	Hypothyroidism, increased intake of vegetables containing carotene
	Decreased visibility of oxy-hemoglobin	Generalized	Anemia, chronic renal disease
Blue	Increased unsat-urated hemo-globin secondary to hypoxia	Lips, mouth, nail beds	Cardiovascular and pulmonary diseases

TECHNIQUE	FINDINGS
■ *Thickness*	**EXPECTED:** Thickness variations, with eyelids thinnest, areas of rubbing thickest. Calluses on hands and feet.
	UNEXPECTED: Atrophy. Hyperkeratosis.
■ *Symmetry*	**EXPECTED:** Bilateral symmetry.
■ *Hygiene*	**EXPECTED:** Clean.

Palpate skin

TECHNIQUE	FINDINGS
■ *Moisture*	**EXPECTED:** Minimal perspiration or oiliness. Increased perspiration (associated with activity, environment, obesity, anxiety, excitement) noticeable on palms, scalp, forehead, axillae.
	UNEXPECTED: Damp intertriginous areas.
■ *Temperature* Palpate with dorsal surface of hand or fingers.	**EXPECTED:** Cool to warm. Bilateral symmetry.
■ *Texture*	**EXPECTED:** Smooth, soft, and even. Roughness resulting from heavy clothing, cold weather, or soap.
	UNEXPECTED: Extensive or widespread roughness.
■ *Turgor and mobility* Gently pinch skin on forearm or in sternal area and release.	**EXPECTED:** Resilience.
	UNEXPECTED: Failure of skin to return to place quickly.

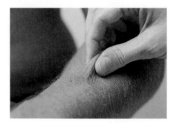

TECHNIQUE   FINDINGS

Inspect and palpate lesions

- *Size*
  Measure all dimensions.
- *Shape*
- *Color*
  Use Wood's lamp to distin-
  guish fluorescing lesions.
- *Blanching*
- *Texture*
  Transilluminate to determine
  presence of fluid.
- *Elevation/depression*
- *Pedunculation*
- *Exudate*
  Note color, odor, amount,
  and consistency of lesion.
- *Configuration*
  Check lesion for annular,
  grouped, linear, arciform, or
  diffuse arrangement.
- *Location/distribution*
  Check lesion for
  generalized/localized, body
  region, patterns, or
  discrete/confluent.

UNEXPECTED: See table on
pp. 32-37.

Hair

Inspect hair over entire body

- *Color*

EXPECTED: Light blond to
black and gray, with alterations
caused by rinses, dyes, and per-
manents.

- *Distribution/quantity*

EXPECTED: Hair present on
scalp, lower face, neck, nares,
ears, chest, axillae, back and
shoulders, arms, legs, pubic areas,
and around nipples. Scalp hair
loss in adult men, adrenal andro-
genic female-pattern alopecia in
adult women.

Primary Skin Lesions

Description	Examples

Macule

Flat, circumscribed area that is a change in skin color; less than 1 cm in diameter

Freckles, flat moles (nevi), petechiae, measles, scarlet fever

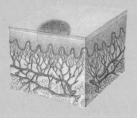

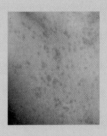

Measles.
From Habif, 1996.

Papule

Elevated, firm, circumscribed area less than 1 cm in diameter

Wart (verruca), elevated moles, lichen planus

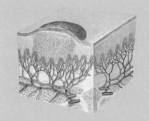

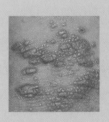

Lichen planus.
From Weston, Lane, Morelli, 1996.

Primary Skin Lesions—cont'd

Description	Examples

Patch

Flat, nonpalpable, irregular-shaped macule more than 1 cm in diameter

Vitiligo, port-wine stains, mongolian spots, café au lait spots

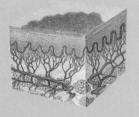

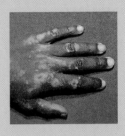

Vitiligo.
From Weston, Lane, and Morelli, 1991.

Plaque

Elevated, firm, and rough lesion with flat top surface greater than 1 cm in diameter

Psoriasis, seborrheic and actinic keratoses

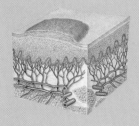

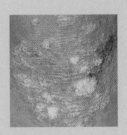

Plaque.
From Habif, 1996.

Continued.

Primary Skin Lesions—cont'd

Description	Examples

Wheal

Elevated irregular-shaped area of cutaneous edema; solid, transient; variable diameter

Insect bites, urticaria, allergic reaction

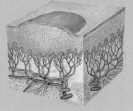

Wheal.
From Farrar et al, 1992.

Nodule

Elevated, firm, circumscribed lesion; deeper in dermis than a papule; 1 to 2 cm in diameter

Erythema nodosum, lipomas

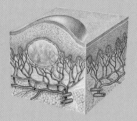

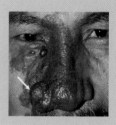

Hypertrophic nodule.
From Goldman and Fitzpatrick, 1999.

Primary Skin Lesions—cont'd

Description	Examples

Tumor

Elevated and solid lesion; may or may not be clearly demarcated; deeper in dermis; greater than 2 cm in diameter

Neoplasms, benign tumor, lipoma, hemangioma

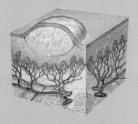

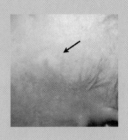

Hemangioma.
From Weston, Lane, Morelli, 1996.

Vesicle

Elevated, circumscribed, superficial, not into dermis; filled with serous fluid; less than 1 cm in diameter

Varicella (chickenpox), herpes zoster (shingles)

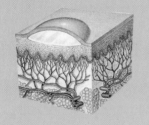

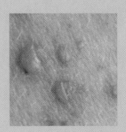

Vesicles caused by varicella.
From Farrar et al, 1992.

Continued.

Primary Skin Lesions—cont'd

Description	Examples

Bulla

Vesicle greater than 1 cm in diameter

Blister, pemphigus vulgaris

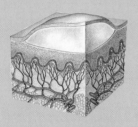

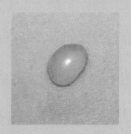

Blister.
From White, 1994.

Pustule

Elevated, superficial lesion; similar to a vesicle but filled with purulent fluid

Impetigo, acne

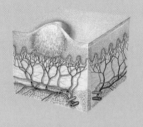

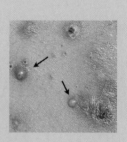

Acne.
From Weston, Lane, Morelli, 1996.

Primary Skin Lesions—cont'd

Description	Examples

Cyst

Elevated, circumscribed, encapsulated lesion; in dermis or subcutaneous layer; filled with liquid or semisolid material

Sebaceous cyst, cystic acne

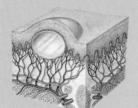

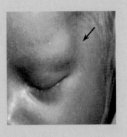

Sebaceous cyst.
From Weston, Lane, Morelli, 1996.

Telangiectasia

Fine, irregular red lines produced by capillary dilation

Telangiectasia in rosacea

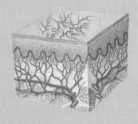

Telangiectasia.
From Lemmi, Lemmi, 2000.

TECHNIQUE	FINDINGS
	UNEXPECTED: Localized or generalized hair loss, inflammation, or scarring. Broken/absent hair shafts. Hirsutism in women.
Palpate for texture	
	EXPECTED: Coarse or fine, curly or straight, shiny, smooth, and resilient. Fine vellus covering body; coarse terminal hair on scalp, on pubis, on axillary areas, and in male beard.
	UNEXPECTED: Dryness and brittleness.

Nails

Inspect nails

- *Color*

  EXPECTED: Variations of pink with varying opacity. Pigment deposits in persons with dark skin. White spots.

  UNEXPECTED: Yellow or green-black discoloration. Diffuse darkening. Pigment deposits in persons with light skin. Longitudinal red, brown, or white streaks or white bands. White, yellow, or green tinge.

- *Length/configuration/ symmetry*

  EXPECTED: Varying shape, smooth and flat/slightly convex, with edges smooth and rounded.

  UNEXPECTED: Jagged, broken, or bitten edges or cuticles. Peeling. Absence of nail.

- *Cleanliness*

  EXPECTED: Clean and neat.

  UNEXPECTED: Unkempt.

- *Ridging and beading*

  EXPECTED: Longitudinal ridging and beading.

TECHNIQUE

FINDINGS

UNEXPECTED: Longitudinal ridging and grooving with lichen planus. Transverse grooving, rippling, and depressions. Pitting.

Palpate nail plate

■ *Texture/firmness/thickness/ uniformity*

EXPECTED: Hard and smooth with uniform thickness.
UNEXPECTED: Thickening or thinning.

■ *Adherence to nail bed*
Gently squeeze between thumb and finger.

EXPECTED: Firmness.
UNEXPECTED: Separation. Boggy nail base.

Measure nail base angle

Inspect fingers when patient places dorsal surfaces of fingertips together.

EXPECTED: 160-degree angle.
UNEXPECTED: Clubbing.

Inspect and palpate proximal and lateral nail fold

UNEXPECTED: Redness, swelling, pus, warts, cysts, tumors, and pain.

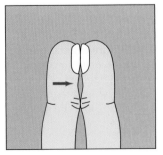

Expected finding.

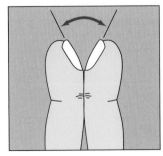

Clubbing.

AIDS TO DIFFERENTIAL DIAGNOSIS

ABNORMALITY	DESCRIPTION
Corn (clavus)	Flat or slightly elevated, circumscribed, painful lesions. Smooth, hard surface. Soft corns—whitish thickenings. Hard corns—sharply delineated, conical.
Callus	Superficial area of hyperkeratosis. Less demarcated than corns. Usually nontender.
Tinea (dermatophytosis)	Papular, pustular, vesicular, erythematous, or scaling lesions. Possible secondary bacterial infection.
Basal cell carcinoma	Cutaneous neoplasm in nodular, pigmented, cystic, sclerosing, superficial, and other forms.
Kaposi sarcoma	Soft, vascular, bluish purple, painless lesions. Macular or papular. May appear as plaques, keloids, or ecchymotic areas.
Eczematous dermatitis	Acute—erythematous, pruritic, weeping vesicles, often excoriated and crusted from scratching. Subacute—erythema and scaling, possible itching. Chronic—thick, lichenified, pruritic plaques.
Paronychia	Redness, swelling, tenderness at lateral and proximal nail folds. Possible purulent drainage under cuticle. Acute or chronic (with nail rippling).
Ingrown nail	Pain and swelling resulting from nail piercing fold and growing into dermis.

PEDIATRIC VARIATIONS
EXAMINATION

TECHNIQUE	FINDINGS

Skin

Inspect hands and feet of newborns for skin creases

EXPECTED: Number of creases is indication of maturity of newborn; the greater the gestational age, the more creases.

UNEXPECTED: Single transverse crease across palm frequently seen in infants with Down syndrome.

AIDS TO DIFFERENTIAL DIAGNOSIS

ABNORMALITY	DESCRIPTION
Café au lait spots	Coffee-colored multiple patches, diameter more than 1 cm.
Seborrheic dermatitis	Thick, yellow, adherent crusted scalp, ear, or neck lesions.
Impetigo	Honey-colored crusted or ruptured vesicles.
Miliaria ("prickly heat")	Irregular, red, macular rash.
Reddened patches	Irregular reddened areas suggestive of richer capillary bed. Include strawberry hemangioma and cavernous hemangioma.
Chickenpox (varicella)	Fever, mild malaise, and pruritic maculopapular skin eruption that becomes vesicular in a matter of hours.
German measles (rubella)	Generalized light pink to red maculopapular rash, low-grade fever, coryza, sore throat, cough.

SAMPLE DOCUMENTATION

Subjective. An 18-year-old female with a body rash. First noticed the rash 4 days ago. Thinks it may be from drinking new citrus juice. Describes rash as red and itchy, with transient bumps on face, neck, arms, legs, torso. No known food allergies. Denied exposure to new contact irritants. No new medications; is currently taking antihistamine for allergic rhinitis. Denies respiratory difficulty, difficulty swallowing, edema. Denies fever, cough, malaise.

Objective. *Skin:* Dark pink maculopapular lesions on face, torso, extremities; large urticarial wheal on right cheek. No excoriation or secondary infection. Turgor resilient. Skin uniformly warm and dry. No edema.

Hair: Curly, black, thick with female distribution pattern. Texture coarse.

Nails: Opaque, short, well-groomed, uniform and without deformities. Nail bed pink. Nail base angle 160 degrees. No redness, exudates, or swelling in surrounding folds and no tenderness to palpation.

5

Lymphatic System

EQUIPMENT

- Centimeter ruler
- Skin-marking pencil

EXAMINATION

Lymphatic system is examined by inspection and palpation, region by region, during the examination of other body systems, as well as with palpation of the spleen.

Lymph Nodes Most Accessible to Inspection and Palpation

Obviously, the more superficial the node, the more accessible it is.

"Necklace" of Nodes
Parotid and retropharyngeal
　　(tonsillar)
Submandibular
Submental
Sublingual (facial)
Superficial anterior cervical
Superficial posterior cervical
Preauricular and postauricular
Occipital
Supraclavicular

Arms
Axillary
Epitrochlear (cubital)

Legs
Superficial superior inguinal
Superficial inferior inguinal
Occasionally, popliteal

TECHNIQUE   FINDINGS

Head and Neck

Inspect visible nodes

Ask if patient is aware of any
lumps.

UNEXPECTED: Edema, erythema, red streaks, or lesions.

Palpate superficial nodes; note size, consistency, mobility, tenderness,
warmth

Bend patient's head slightly
forward or to side. Palpate
gently with pads of second,
third, fourth fingers.

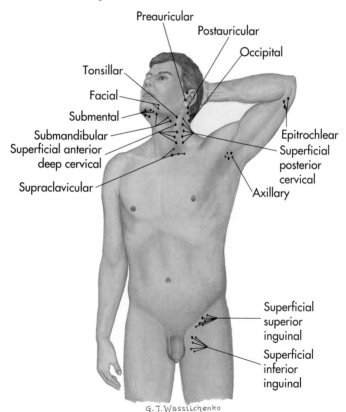

Preauricular

Postauricular

Occipital

Tonsillar

Facial

Submental

Submandibular

Superficial anterior
deep cervical

Supraclavicular

Epitrochlear

Superficial
posterior
cervical

Axillary

Superficial
superior
inguinal

Superficial
inferior
inguinal

G.J.Wassilchenko

TECHNIQUE   FINDINGS

Head/Neck

- *Occipital nodes at base of skull*
- *Postauricular nodes over mastoid process*
- *Preauricular nodes in front of ears*
- *Parotid and retropharyngeal nodes at angle of mandible*
- *Submandibular nodes between angle and tip of mandible*
- *Submental nodes behind tip of mandible*

EXPECTED: Nodes accessible to palpation but not large or firm enough to be felt.
UNEXPECTED: Enlarged, tender, red or discolored, fixed, matted, inflamed, or warm nodes, increased vascularity.

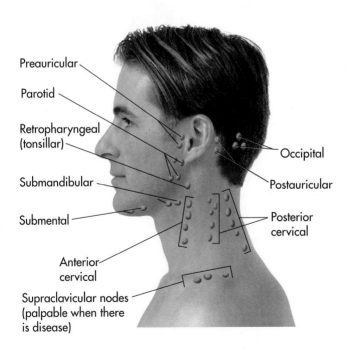

Preauricular

Parotid

Retropharyngeal (tonsillar)

Submandibular

Submental

Anterior cervical

Supraclavicular nodes (palpable when there is disease)

Occipital

Postauricular

Posterior cervical

TECHNIQUE   FINDINGS

Neck

- *Superficial cervical nodes at sternocleidomastoid*
- *Posterior cervical nodes along anterior border of trapezius*
- *Deep cervical nodes along anterior border of trapezius*
- *Supraclavicular areas*
  If enlarged nodes are found, inspect regions drained by nodes for infection or malignancy and examine other regions for enlargement.

EXPECTED: Nodes accessible to palpation but not large or firm enough to be felt.
UNEXPECTED: Enlarged, tender, red or discolored, fixed, matted, inflamed, or warm nodes, increased vascularity.
UNEXPECTED: Detection of Virchow nodes.

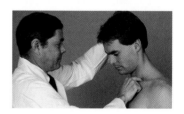

Axillae

Inspect visible nodes

Ask if patient is aware of any lumps.

UNEXPECTED: Edema, erythema, red streaks, or lesions.

Palpate superficial nodes for size, consistency, mobility, tenderness, warmth

Using firm, deliberate, gentle touch, rotate fingertips and palm. Attempt to glide fingers beneath nodes.

Axillary nodes

Support patient's forearm with your contralateral arm, and bring palm of examining hand flat into axilla.
If enlarged nodes are found, inspect regions drained by nodes for infection or malignancy, and examine other regions for enlargement.

EXPECTED: Nodes accessible to palpation but not large or firm enough to be felt.
UNEXPECTED: Enlarged, tender, red or discolored, fixed, matted, inflamed, or warm nodes, increased vascularity.

TECHNIQUE	FINDINGS

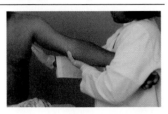

Other Lymph Nodes

Inspect visible nodes

Ask if patient is aware of any lumps.

UNEXPECTED: Edema, erythema, red streaks, or lesions.

Palpate superficial nodes for size, consistency, mobility, tenderness, warmth

Systematically palpate other areas, moving hand in circular fashion, probing without pressing hard.

EXPECTED: Nodes accessible to palpation but not large or firm enough to be felt.
UNEXPECTED: Enlarged, tender, red or discolored, fixed, matted, inflamed, or warm nodes, increased vascularity.

- *Epitrochlear nodes*
  Support elbow in one hand while exploring with other.

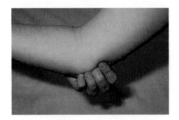

TECHNIQUE   FINDINGS

- *Inguinal and popliteal area*
  Have patient lie supine with
  knee slightly flexed.

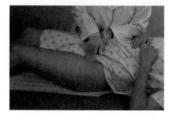

If enlarged nodes are found,
inspect regions drained by
nodes for infection or malignancy and examine other regions for enlargement.

AIDS TO DIFFERENTIAL DIAGNOSIS

ABNORMALITY	DESCRIPTION
Acute lymphangitis	Pain, malaise, illness, possibly fever. Red streak (tracing of fine lines) may follow course of lymphatic collecting duct. Inflamed area sometimes slightly indurated and palpable to gentle touch. Related infection possible distally, particularly interdigitally.
Non-Hodgkin lymphoma	Well-defined, solid neoplasm, often in lymph nodes or spleen.
Hodgkin disease	Painless, inexorably progressive enlargement of cervical lymph nodes. Generally asymmetric. Nodes sometimes matted and generally very firm, almost rubbery. Nodes sometimes produce pressure on surrounding structures, prompting need for medical care.

ABNORMALITY	DESCRIPTION
Epstein-Barr virus; mono-nucleosis	Pharyngitis, fever, fatigue, malaise. Frequently spleno-megaly and/or rash. Palpable nodes generalized but more commonly in anterior and posterior cervical chains. Nodes vary in firmness, are generally discrete, are occasionally tender.
Streptococcal pharyngitis	Sore throat. Often runny nose. Sometimes headache, fatigue, abdominal pain. Firm, discrete, often tender anterior cervical nodes generally felt.
Herpes simplex	Often discrete labial and gingival ulcers, high fever, enlargement of anterior cervical and submandibular nodes. Nodes tend to be firm, quite discrete, movable, tender.
Acquired immunodeficiency syndrome (AIDS)	Recurrent, often severe, opportunistic infections. Initially lymphadenopathy, fatigue, fever, weight loss.
Human immunodeficiency virus (HIV) seropositivity	Warning signs: severe fatigue, malaise, weakness, persistent unexplained weight loss, persistent lymphadenopathy, fevers, arthralgias, persistent diarrhea.

Some Conditions Simulating Lymph Node Enlargement

Lymphangioma
Hemangioma (tends to feel spongy; appears reddish blue, depending on size and extent of angiomatous involvement)
Branchial cleft cyst (sometimes accompanied by tiny orifice in neck on line extending to ear)
Thyroglossal duct cyst
Laryngocele
Esophageal diverticulum
Thyroid goiter
Graves disease
Hashimoto thyroiditis
Parotid swelling (e.g., from mumps or tumor)

PEDIATRIC VARIATIONS
EXAMINATION

TECHNIQUE	FINDINGS

Head and Neck
Palpate superficial nodes
- *Occipital nodes at base of skull*
- *Postauricular nodes over mastoid process*

EXPECTED: In children, small, firm, discrete, nontender, nonmovable nodes in occipital, postauricular chains.

Other Lymph Nodes
Palpate superficial nodes
- *Inguinal and popliteal area*

EXPECTED: In children, small, firm, discrete nodes; nontender, movable in inguinal chain.

SAMPLE DOCUMENTATION

Subjective. A 25-year-old woman complains of difficulty swallowing and sore throat for 3 days, now subsiding. Fever to 38° C (100.5° F) for 2 days. Has been using aspirin and throat lozenges for pain relief.
Objective. No visible enlargement of lymph nodes in any area. Enlarged node (2 cm in diameter) palpated in left posterior cervical triangle; firm, nontender, movable, no overlying warmth, erythema, or edema. A few shotty nodes palpated in posterior cervical triangles bilaterally and in femoral chains bilaterally.

6

Head and Neck

EQUIPMENT

- Tape measure
- Stethoscope
- Cup of water
- Transilluminator

EXAMINATION

Ask patient to sit.

TECHNIQUE	FINDINGS
Head and Face	
Observe head position	**EXPECTED:** Upright, midline, still. **UNEXPECTED:** Horizontal jerking or bobbing, nodding, tilted.
Inspect facial features	
■ *Shape* Observe eyelids, eyebrows, palpebral fissures, nasolabial folds, mouth at rest, during movement, with expression.	**EXPECTED:** Variations according to race, sex, age, body build. **UNEXPECTED:** Change in shape. Unusual features: Edema, puffiness, coarsened features, prominent eyes, hirsutism, lack of expression, excessive perspiration, pallor, or pigmentation variations. Tics.

TECHNIQUE	FINDINGS

- *Symmetry*
  Note if asymmetry affects all features of one side or a portion of face.

EXPECTED: Slight asymmetry.
UNEXPECTED: Facial nerve paralysis, facial nerve weakness, or problem with peripheral trigeminal nerve.

- *Characteristic facies*

Inspect skull and scalp

- *Size/shape/symmetry*

EXPECTED: Symmetric.

- *Scalp condition*
  Systematically part hair from frontal to occipital region.

UNEXPECTED: Lesions, scabs, tenderness, parasites, nits, scaliness.

- *Hair pattern*
  Pay special attention to areas behind ears, at hairline, at crown.

EXPECTED: Bitemporal recession or balding over crown in men.
UNEXPECTED: Random areas of alopecia.

Palpate head and scalp

- *Symmetry*
  Palpate in gentle, rotary motion from front to back.

EXPECTED: Symmetric and smooth with bones indistinguishable. Ridge of sagittal fissure occasionally palpable.
UNEXPECTED: Indentations or depressions.

Palpate hair

- *Texture/color distribution*

EXPECTED: Smooth, symmetrically distributed.
UNEXPECTED: Splitting or cracked ends. Coarse, dry, or brittle. Fine and silky.

Palpate temporal arteries

  Note course of arteries.

UNEXPECTED: Thickening, hardness, or tenderness.

TECHNIQUE	FINDINGS

Auscultate temporal arteries and over skull and eyes

EXPECTED: No bruits.

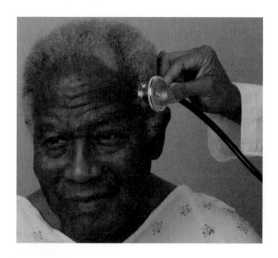

Inspect salivary glands

- *Symmetry/size*
  Palpate if asymmetry noted. Have patient open mouth and press on salivary duct to attempt to express material.

UNEXPECTED: Asymmetry or enlargement. Tenderness. Discrete nodule.

Neck

Inspect neck

- *Symmetry*
  Inspect in usual position, in slight hyperextension, and during swallowing. Look for landmarks of anterior and posterior triangles.

EXPECTED: Bilateral symmetry of sternocleidomastoid and trapezius muscles.
UNEXPECTED: Asymmetry, torticollis.

- *Trachea*
  Inspect in usual position, in slight hyperextension, and while patient swallows.

EXPECTED: Midline placement.

TECHNIQUE

FINDINGS

- *Condition of neck*

UNEXPECTED: Masses, webbing, excessive posterior skinfolds, unusually short neck, distention of jugular vein, prominence of carotid arteries, or edema.

Evaluate range of motion

Have patient flex, extend, rotate, laterally turn head and neck.

EXPECTED: Smooth.
UNEXPECTED: Pain, dizziness, or limitation of motion.

Palpate neck

- *Trachea*
Place thumb on each side of trachea in lower portion of neck, and compare space between trachea and sternocleidomastoid on each side.

EXPECTED: Midline position.
UNEXPECTED: Deviation to right or left.

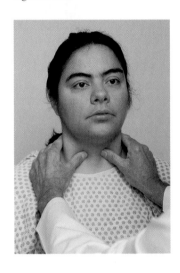

- *Hyoid bone/thyroid and cricoid cartilages*
Have patient swallow.

EXPECTED: Smooth. Moves during swallowing.
UNEXPECTED: Tender.

TECHNIQUE	FINDINGS

■ *Cartilaginous rings of trachea*
Have patient swallow.

EXPECTED: Distinct.
UNEXPECTED: Tender.

■ *Tracheal tug*
With neck extended, palpate for movement with index finger and thumb on each side of trachea below thyroid isthmus.

UNEXPECTED: Tug synchronous with pulse.

Palpate lymph nodes

■ *Size/consistency, mobility/condition*

UNEXPECTED: Enlarged, matted, tender, fixed, warm.

Palpate thyroid gland

■ *Symmetry*
Observe from frontal and lateral positions while patient hyperextends neck. Then observe as patient sips water while neck is hyperextended.

UNEXPECTED: Asymmetry. Enlarged and visible thyroid gland.

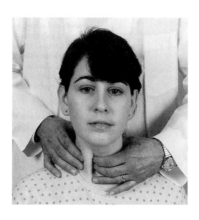

TECHNIQUE	FINDINGS
■ *Size/shape/configuration/ consistency*	
Stand either facing or behind patient. Have patient hold head slightly forward and tipped toward side being examined. Lightly palpate isthmus and lateral lobes. Give water to patient to facilitate swallowing.	**EXPECTED:** Lobes (if felt) small and smooth. Gland rises freely with swallowing. Right lobe as much as 25% larger than left. Tissue firm and pliable.
	UNEXPECTED: Enlarged, tender nodules (smooth or irregular, soft or hard); coarse tissue; gritty sensation.
If gland is enlarged, auscultate for vascular sounds with stethoscope bell.	**UNEXPECTED:** Bruit.

AIDS TO DIFFERENTIAL DIAGNOSIS

ABNORMALITY	DESCRIPTION
Myxedema	Dull, puffy, yellow skin. Coarse, sparse hair. Temporal loss of eyebrows. Periorbital edema. Prominent tongue. Hypothyroidism (see table on p. 57).
Graves disease	Diffuse thyroid enlargement, hyperthyroidism. Various pathologic conditions—ophthalmologic (prominent eyes, lid retraction, staring or startled expression), dermatologic (fine and moist skin, fine hair), musculoskeletal (muscle weakness), cardiac (tachycardia) (see table on p. 57).
Down syndrome	Depressed nasal bridge, epicanthal folds, mongoloid slant of eyes, low-set ears, large tongue.

Hyperthyroidism Versus Hypothyroidism

System or Structure Affected	Hyperthyroidism	Hypothyroidism
Constitutional		
Temperature preference	Cool climate	Warm climate
Weight	Loss	Gain
Emotional state	Nervous, easily irritated, highly energetic	Lethargic, complacent, uninterested
Hair	Fine, with hair loss; failure to hold permanent wave	Coarse, with tendency to break
Skin	Warm, fine, hyperpigmentation at pressure points	Coarse, scaling, dry
Fingernails	Thin, with tendency to break; may show onycholysis	Thick
Eyes	Bilateral or unilateral proptosis, lid retraction, double vision	Puffiness in periorbital region
Neck	Goiter, change in shirt neck size, pain over thyroid	No goiter
Cardiac	Tachycardia, arrhythmia, palpitations	No change noted
Gastrointestinal	Increased frequency of bowel movements; diarrhea rare	Constipation
Menstrual	Scant flow, amenorrhea	Menorrhagia
Neuromuscular	Increasing weakness, especially of proximal muscles	Lethargic, but good muscular strength

Headaches

Headaches are one of the most common complaints and probably one of the most self-medicated. They are not always benign. A history of insistent headache that is severe and recurrent must always be given attention. Sometimes the underlying cause is life threatening, such as a brain tumor. Sometimes it is life intimidating, such as migraines. At other times it is easily confronted, such as when it is the result of drinking wine. The patient's history is fully as important as the physical examination in getting at the root of a headache. Various kinds of headaches can be compared as follows.

Characteristic	Classic Migraine	Common Migraine	Cluster	Hypertensive	Muscular, Tension	Temporal Arteritis
Age at onset	Childhood	Childhood	Adulthood	Adulthood	Adulthood	Older adulthood
Location	Unilateral	Generalized	Unilateral	Bilateral or occipital	Unilateral or bilateral	Unilateral or bilateral
Duration	Hours to days	Hours to days	½ to 2 hours	Hours	Hours to days	Hours to days
Time of onset	Morning or night	Morning or night	Night	Morning	Anytime, commonly in afternoon or evening	Anytime
Quality of pain	Pulsating or throbbing	Pulsating or throbbing	Intense burning, boring, searing, knifelike	Throbbing	Bandlike, constricting	Throbbing

Prodromal event	Well-defined neurologic event, scotoma, aphasia, hemianopsia, aura	Vague neurologic changes, personality change, fluid retention, appetite loss	None	None	None	None
Precipitating event	Menstrual period, missing meals, birth control pills, letdown after stress	Menstrual period, missing meals, birth control pills, letdown after stress	None	Alcohol consumption	Stress, anger, bruxism	None
Frequency	Twice a week	Twice a week	Daily	Several times nightly for several nights, then none	Daily	Daily
Gender predilection	Females	Females	Equal	Males	Equal	Equal
Other symptoms	Nausea, vomiting	Nausea, vomiting	Generally remits as day progresses	Increased lacrimation, nasal discharge	None	None

PEDIATRIC VARIATIONS

EXAMINATION

TECHNIQUE	FINDINGS

Head and Face

Palpate head and scalp

- *Symmetry*

EXPECTED: An infant's head circumference is 2 cm greater than chest circumference up to the age of 2 years.

  In infants, transilluminate skull

EXPECTED: 2-cm ring of light.

- *Skull condition*

EXPECTED: In infants, posterior fontanels closed at 2 months; anterior fontanels closed at 18 to 24 months.
UNEXPECTED: Tenderness or depressions; sunken areas; swelling, bulging, or depressed fontanels.

- *Scalp*

EXPECTED: Free movement.
UNEXPECTED: Fixation of scalp, bulging either on one side or crossing midline of scalp.

Percuss skull

EXPECTED: Macewen sign, cracked-pot sound, is physiologic when fontanels are open.
UNEXPECTED: Macewen sign may indicate increased intracranial pressure after fontanel closure.

Auscultate temporal arteries and over skull and eyes

EXPECTED: Bruits are common in children up to age 5 years.

TECHNIQUE	FINDINGS
Neck Palpate thyroid gland	
■ *Symmetry*	**EXPECTED:** In children, thyroid gland may be palpable. **UNEXPECTED:** Tenderness.

SAMPLE DOCUMENTATION

Head. Held erect and midline. Skull normocephalic, symmetric, smooth without deformities. Facial features symmetric. No frontal or maxillary sinus tenderness elicited with palpation or percussion. Salivary glands not inflamed or tender. Temporal artery pulsations visible bilaterally, soft and nontender to palpation. No bruits.

Neck. Trachea midline. No jugular venous distention (JVD) or carotid artery prominence. Thyroid palpable, firm, smooth, not enlarged. Thyroid and cartilages move with swallowing. No nodules or tenderness. No bruits. Full range of motion (ROM) of neck without discomfort.

Clinical and Reference Notes

7

Eyes

EQUIPMENT

- Snellen chart or E chart
- Eye cover, gauze, or opaque card
- Rosenbaum or Jaeger near-vision card
- Penlight
- Cotton wisp
- Ophthalmoscope

EXAMINATION

Ask patient to sit or stand.

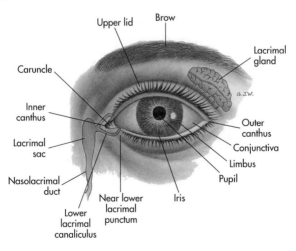

TECHNIQUE   FINDINGS

Visual Testing

Measure visual acuity in each eye separately

- *Distance vision*
  Use Snellen chart or **E** chart.
  If testing with and without
  corrective lenses, test without
  lenses first and record readings separately.
- *Near vision*
  Use near-vision card.
- *Peripheral vision*
  Test nasal, temporal, superior,
  inferior fields by moving
  your finger into field from
  outside.

EXPECTED: Vision 20/20 with
or without lenses with near and
far vision in each eye.
UNEXPECTED: Myopia, am-
blyopia, or presbyopia.

UNEXPECTED: Fields of vision
more limited than 60 degrees
nasally, 90 degrees temporally,
50 degrees superiorly, 70 degrees inferiorly.

External Examination

Inspect eyebrows

- *Size/extension*

EXPECTED: Unusually thin if
plucked.
UNEXPECTED: End short of
temporal canthus.

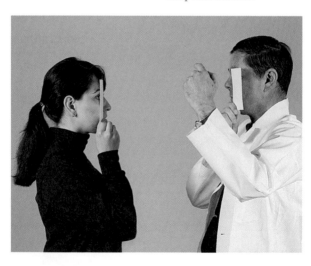

TECHNIQUE	FINDINGS
■ *Hair texture*	**UNEXPECTED:** Coarse.
Inspect orbital area	
	UNEXPECTED: Edema, puffiness not related to aging, or sagging tissue below orbit. Xanthelasma.
Inspect eyelids	
■ *Eyelid position*	**UNEXPECTED:** Ectropion or
■ *Ability to open wide and close completely* Examine with eyes lightly closed, closed tightly, open wide.	entropion. **EXPECTED:** Superior eyelid covering a portion of iris when open. **UNEXPECTED:** Fasciculations when lightly closed. Ptosis. Lagophthalmos.
■ *Eyelid margin*	**UNEXPECTED:** Flakiness, redness, or swelling. Hordeola.
■ *Eyelashes*	**EXPECTED:** Present on both lids. Turned outward.
Palpate eyelids	
	UNEXPECTED: Nodules.
Palpate eye	
	EXPECTED: Can be gently pushed into orbit without discomfort. **UNEXPECTED:** Firm and resists palpation.
Pull down lower lids and inspect conjunctivae and sclerae	
■ *Color* Inspect upper tarsal conjunctivae only if presence of foreign body is suspected.	**EXPECTED:** Conjunctivae clear and inapparent. Sclerae white and visible above irides only when eyelids are wide open.

TECHNIQUE	FINDINGS
	UNEXPECTED: Conjunctivae with erythema. Sclerae yellow or green. Sclerae with dark, rust-colored pigment anterior to insertion of medial rectus muscle.
■ *Condition*	**UNEXPECTED:** Exudate. Pterygium. Corneal arcus senilis or opacities.

Inspect lacrimal gland region

■ *Lacrimal gland puncta*
Palpate lower orbital rim near inner canthus. If temporal aspect of upper lid feels full, evert lid and inspect gland.

EXPECTED: Slight elevations with central depression on both upper and lower lid margins.
UNEXPECTED: Enlarged glands. Dry eyes.

Test corneal sensitivity

Touch wisp of cotton to cornea.

EXPECTED: Bilateral blink reflex.

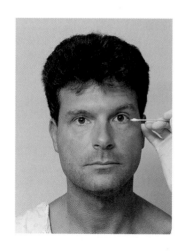

TECHNIQUE	FINDINGS

Inspect external eyes

- *Corneal clarity*
  Shine light tangentially on cornea.

  UNEXPECTED: Blood vessels present.

- *Irides*

  EXPECTED: Clearly visible pattern. Similar color.

- *Pupillary size/shape*

  EXPECTED: Round, regular, equal in size.

  UNEXPECTED: Miosis, mydriasis, anisocoria, or coloboma.

- *Pupillary response to light*

  EXPECTED: Constricting with consensual response of opposite pupil.

- *Pupillary accommodation*

  EXPECTED: Constricting when pupils focus on near object or dilating when focus changes from near to distant.

Extraocular Eye Muscles

Evaluate muscle balance and movement of eyes

- *Six cardinal fields of gaze*
  Hold patient's chin, and ask patient to watch finger or penlight.

  EXPECTED: A few horizontal nystagmic beats. Smooth, full, coordinated movement of eyes.

  UNEXPECTED: Sustained or jerking nystagmus. Exposure of sclera from lid lag. Inability of eye to move in all directions.

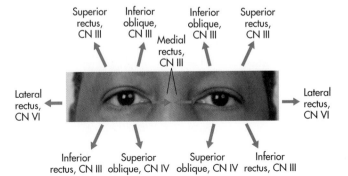

Superior rectus, CN III | Inferior oblique, CN III | Medial rectus, CN III | Inferior oblique, CN III | Superior rectus, CN III

Lateral rectus, CN VI | Lateral rectus, CN VI

Inferior rectus, CN III | Superior oblique, CN IV | Superior oblique, CN IV | Inferior rectus, CN III

TECHNIQUE   FINDINGS

- *Corneal light reflex*
  Direct light at nasal bridge
  from 30 cm (12 inches). Have
  patient look at nearby object.

  EXPECTED: Light reflected
  symmetrically from both eyes.

- *Cover-uncover test*
  Perform if imbalance found
  with corneal light reflex test.
  Have patient stare ahead at
  near, fixed object. Cover one
  eye and observe other; remove cover and observe uncovered eye. Repeat with
  other eye.

  UNEXPECTED: Movement of
  covered or uncovered eye.

Ophthalmoscopic Examination

Inspect internal eye

- *Lens clarity*
- *Anterior chamber*
  Shine focused light tangentially at limbus. Note illumi-
  nation of iris nasally.

  UNEXPECTED: Shallow chamber. If observed, avoid mydri-
  atics.

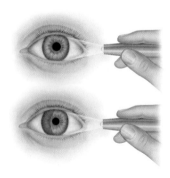

TECHNIQUE	FINDINGS

■ *Use ophthalmoscope*
With patient looking at distant object, direct light at pupil from about 30 cm (12 inches). Move toward patient, observing:
  ▪ *Red reflex*
  ▪ *Fundus*

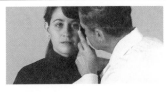

UNEXPECTED: Opacities.
EXPECTED: Yellow or pink background, depending on race. Possible crescents or dots of pigment at disc margin, usually temporally.
UNEXPECTED: Discrete areas of pigmentation away from disc. Lesions. Drusen bodies. Hemorrhages.

■ *Blood vessel characteristics*
Follow blood vessels distally in each quadrant, noting crossings of arterioles and venules.

EXPECTED: Possible venous pulsations (should be documented). Arteriole/venule (A/V) ratio 3:5 or 2:3.
UNEXPECTED: Glaucomatous cupping, nicking, crossing, tortuosity.

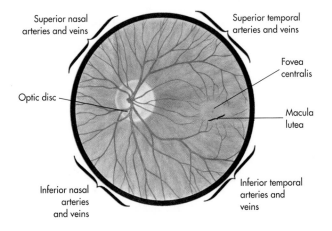

Superior nasal arteries and veins

Superior temporal arteries and veins

Fovea centralis

Optic disc

Macula lutea

Inferior nasal arteries and veins

Inferior temporal arteries and veins

TECHNIQUE	FINDINGS
■ *Disc characteristics*	**EXPECTED:** Yellow to creamy pink, varying by race. Sharp, well-defined margin, especially in temporal region; 1.5 mm diameter. **UNEXPECTED:** Myelinated nerve fibers. Papilledema. Glaucomatous cupping.
■ *Macula densa characteristics* Ask patient to look directly at light.	**EXPECTED:** Yellow dot surrounded by deep pink.

AIDS TO DIFFERENTIAL DIAGNOSIS

ABNORMALITY	DESCRIPTION
Strabismus (paralytic and nonparalytic)	Eyes do not focus simultaneously. Can focus separately in nonparalytic type.
Episcleritis	Inflammation of superficial layers of sclera anterior to insertion of rectus muscles. Generally localized with purplish elevation of a few millimeters.
Cataracts	Opacity of lens, generally central, occasionally peripheral.
Diabetic retinopathy (background)	Dot hemorrhages or microaneurysms. Hard exudates (bright yellow, sharply defined borders) and soft exudates (dull yellow spots, poorly defined margins).

PEDIATRIC VARIATIONS

EXAMINATION

TECHNIQUE	FINDINGS

Visual Testing

Measure visual acuity

■ *Distance vision*

Visual acuity is tested, when child is cooperative, with Snellen **E** or picture chart, usually at about 3 years of age.

EXPECTED:

AGE, YEARS	ACUITY
3	20/50
4	20/40
5	20/30
6	20/20

Infants should be able to focus on and track a face or light through 60 degrees.

Extraocular Eye Muscles

Evaluate muscle balance and movement of eyes

Evaluation of six cardinal fields of gaze is performed as with adults. You may, however, need to hold child's head still.

SAMPLE DOCUMENTATION

Eyes. Near vision 20/40 in each eye uncorrected, corrected to 20/20 with glasses. Distant vision 20/20 by Snellen. Visual fields full by confrontation. Extraocular movements intact and full, no nystagmus. Corneal light reflex equal.

Lids and globes symmetric. No ptosis. Eyebrows full, no edema or lesions evident.

Conjunctivae pink, sclerae white. No discharge evident. Cornea clear, corneal reflex intact. Irides brown; pupils equal, round, reactive to light and accommodation.

Ophthalmoscopic examination reveals red reflex. Discs cream colored, borders well defined with temporal pigmentation in both eyes (OU). No venous pulsations evident at disc. Arteriole/venule ratio 3:5; no nicking or crossing changes, hemorrhages, or exudates noted. Maculae are yellow OU.

Clinical and Reference Notes

8

Ears, Nose, and Throat

EQUIPMENT

- Otoscope with pneumatic attachment
- Tuning fork
- Nasal speculum
- Tongue blades
- Gloves
- Gauze
- Penlight, sinus transilluminator, or light from otoscope

EXAMINATION

Have patient sit.

TECHNIQUE   FINDINGS

Ears

Inspect auricles and mastoid area

Examine lateral and medial
surfaces and surrounding tissue.

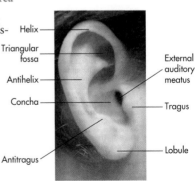

Helix

Triangular
fossa

Antihelix

Concha

Antitragus

External
auditory
meatus

Tragus

Lobule

73

TECHNIQUE	FINDINGS
■ *Size/shape/symmetry*	**EXPECTED**: Familial variations. Auricles of equal size and similar appearance. Darwin tubercle. **UNEXPECTED**: Unequal size or configuration. Cauliflower ear and other deformities.
■ *Lesions*	**UNEXPECTED**: Moles, cysts or other lesions, nodules, or tophi.
■ *Color*	**EXPECTED**: Same color as facial skin. **UNEXPECTED**: Blueness, pallor, or excessive redness.
■ *Position* Draw imaginary line between outer canthus and most prominent protuberance of occiput. Draw imaginary line perpendicular to first line and anterior to auricle.	**EXPECTED**: Top of auricle touching or above line. Vertical position. **UNEXPECTED**: Auricle positioned below line; unequal alignment. Lateral posterior angle greater than 10 degrees.
■ *Preauricular area*	**EXPECTED**: Preauricular pits or smooth skin. **UNEXPECTED**: Openings in preauricular area, discharge.
■ *External auditory canal*	**EXPECTED**: No discharge, no odor; canal walls pink. **UNEXPECTED**: Serous, bloody, or purulent discharge; foul smell.
Palpate auricles and mastoid area	
	EXPECTED: Firm and mobile, readily recoil from folded position; nontender. **UNEXPECTED**: Tenderness, swelling, nodules. Pain from pulling on lobule.

TECHNIQUE   FINDINGS

Inspect auditory canal with otoscope

Tilt patient's head toward opposite shoulder. Pull auricle
upward and back while gently inserting speculum. Assess
canal from meatus to tym-
panic membrane.

EXPECTED: Cerumen in varying color and texture. Pink
canal. Hairs in outer third of
canal.
UNEXPECTED: Cerumen ob-
scures tympanic membrane,
odor, lesions, discharge, scaling,
excessive redness, foreign bodies.

Inspect tympanic membrane

■ *Landmarks*
Vary light direction to observe entire membrane and
annulus.

EXPECTED: Visible umbo,
handle of malleus, light reflex.
UNEXPECTED: Perforations,
landmarks not visible.

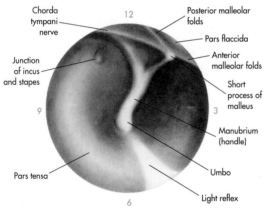

From Barkauskas et al, 2001.

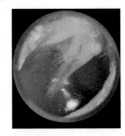

From Barkauskas et al, 2001.

TECHNIQUE	FINDINGS
■ *Color*	**EXPECTED:** Translucent, pearly gray. **UNEXPECTED:** Amber, yellow, blue, deep red, chalky white, dull, white flecks, or dense white plaques; air bubbles or fluid level.
■ *Contour*	**EXPECTED:** Slightly conical with concavity at umbo. **UNEXPECTED:** Bulging (more conical, usually with loss of bony landmarks and distorted light reflex) or retracted (more concave, usually with accentuated bony landmarks and distorted light reflex).
■ *Mobility* Seal canal with speculum, and gently apply positive (squeeze) and negative (release) pressure with pneumatic attachment.	**EXPECTED:** Movement in and out. **UNEXPECTED:** No movement.
Assess hearing	
■ *Questions during history*	**EXPECTED:** Responds to questions appropriately. **UNEXPECTED:** Excessive requests for repetition. Speech with monotonous tone and erratic volume.
■ *Whispered voice* Have patient mask hearing in one ear by moving finger rapidly up and down in ear canal. Stand 1 to 2 feet from other ear and softly whisper one- to two-syllable words. Repeat with untested ear.	**EXPECTED:** Patient repeats words correctly at least 50% of the time. **UNEXPECTED:** Patient unable to repeat whispered words.

TECHNIQUE	FINDINGS

- *Weber test*
  Place base of vibrating tuning fork on midline vertex of head. Repeat with one ear occluded.

EXPECTED: Sound heard equally in both ears (unoccluded). Sound heard better in occluded ear.

UNEXPECTED: See table below.

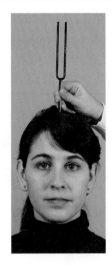

Weber test

Interpretation of Tuning Fork Tests

	Weber Test	Rinne Test
Expected findings	No lateralization but will lateralize to ear occluded by patient	Air conduction heard longer than bone conduction by 2:1 ratio *(Rinne positive)*
Conductive hearing loss	Lateralization to deaf ear unless sensorineural loss	Bone conduction heard longer than air conduction in affected ear *(Rinne negative)*
Sensorineural hearing loss	Lateralization to better-hearing ear unless conductive loss	Air conduction heard longer than bone conduction in affected ear, but less than 2:1 ratio

TECHNIQUE	FINDINGS

- *Rinne test*

  Place base of vibrating tuning fork against mastoid bone, note seconds until sound is no longer heard; then quickly move fork 1 to 2 cm (½ to 1 inch) from auditory canal; and note seconds until sound is no longer heard. Repeat with other ear.

EXPECTED: Measurement of air-conducted sound twice as long as measurement of bone-conducted sound.
UNEXPECTED: See table on p. 77.

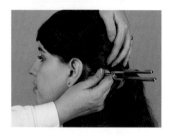 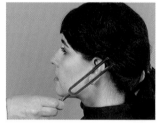

Rinne test

Nose and Sinuses

Inspect external nose

- *Shape/size*

EXPECTED: Smooth. Columella directly midline, width is not greater than diameter of naris.
UNEXPECTED: Swelling or depression of nasal bridge. Transverse crease at junction of nose cartilage and bone.

- *Color*

EXPECTED: Conforms to face color.

- *Nares*

EXPECTED: Oval. Symmetrically positioned.
UNEXPECTED: Asymmetry, discharge, flaring, narrowing.

TECHNIQUE	FINDINGS

Palpate ridge and soft tissues of nose

EXPECTED: Firm and stable structures.
UNEXPECTED: Displacement of bone and cartilage, tenderness, or masses.

Evaluate patency of nares

Occlude one naris with finger on side of nose, ask patient to breathe through nose. Repeat with other naris.

EXPECTED: Noiseless, easy breathing.
UNEXPECTED: Noisy breathing; occlusion.

Inspect nasal mucosa and nasal septum

Tilt patient's head back. Use nasal speculum and strong light. Do no overdilate naris or touch septum.

■ *Color*

EXPECTED: Mucosa deep pink and glistening. Turbinates same color as surrounding area.
UNEXPECTED: Increased redness of mucosa or localized redness and swelling in vestibule. Turbinates bluish gray or pale pink.

■ *Shape*

EXPECTED: Septum close to midline and fairly straight, thicker anteriorly than posteriorly. Inferior and middle turbinates visible.
UNEXPECTED: Asymmetry of posterior nasal cavities, septal deviation.

■ *Condition*

EXPECTED: Possibly film of clear discharge on septum. Possibly hairs in vestibule. Turbinates firm.

TECHNIQUE	FINDINGS

UNEXPECTED: Discharge, bleeding, crusting, masses, or lesions. Swollen, boggy turbinates. Perforated septum. Polyps.

Inspect frontal and maxillary sinus area

UNEXPECTED: Swelling.

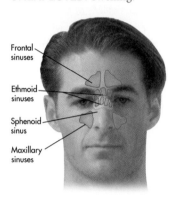

Frontal sinuses

Ethmoid sinuses

Sphenoid sinus

Maxillary sinuses

Palpate frontal and maxillary sinuses

Press thumbs up under bony brow on each side of nose. Palpate with thumbs or index or middle fingers under zygomatic processes.

EXPECTED: Nontender on palpation.
UNEXPECTED: Tenderness or swelling.

Percuss frontal and maxillary sinuses

Lightly tap directly over each sinus area with index finger.

UNEXPECTED: Tenderness, swelling, or pain.

TECHNIQUE   FINDINGS

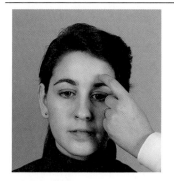
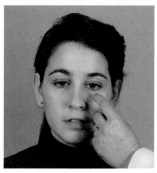

Mouth

Inspect and palpate lips with mouth closed

Have patient remove lipstick
(if applicable).

- *Symmetry*

    EXPECTED: Symmetric verti-
    cally and horizontally at rest
    and moving.
    UNEXPECTED: Asymmetric.

- *Color*

    EXPECTED: Pink, distinct bor-
    der between lips and facial skin.
    UNEXPECTED: Pallor, circum-
    oral pallor, bluish purple, or
    cherry red.

- *Condition*

    EXPECTED: Smooth.
    UNEXPECTED: Dry, cracked;
    swelling, angioedema; cheilosis;
    lesions; plaques; vesicles; nod-
    ules, ulcerations; or round, oval,
    or irregular bluish gray macules.

Inspect teeth

- *Occlusion*
    Have patient clench teeth and
    smile with lips spread.

    EXPECTED: Upper molars in-
    terdigitate with groove on lower
    molars. Premolars and canines
    interdigitate fully. Upper in-
    cisors slightly overriding lower
    incisors.

TECHNIQUE	FINDINGS

UNEXPECTED: Malocclusion. Protrusion of lower incisors. Problems with bite.

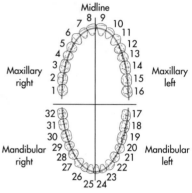

From Miyasaki-Ching, 1997.

■ *Color*

EXPECTED: Ivory, stained yellow or brown.
UNEXPECTED: Discolorations may indicate caries.

■ *Condition*

EXPECTED: 32 teeth, firmly anchored.
UNEXPECTED: Caries and loose or missing teeth.

Inspect buccal mucosa

Have patient remove any dental appliances and then partially open mouth. Use tongue blade and bright light to assess.

■ *Color*

EXPECTED: Pinkish red.
UNEXPECTED: Deeply pigmented. Whitish or pinkish scars.

TECHNIQUE	FINDINGS
■ *Condition*	**EXPECTED:** Smooth and moist. Whitish yellow or whitish pink Stensen duct. Fordyce spots. **UNEXPECTED:** White, round, or oval ulcerative lesions; red spot at opening of Stensen duct.

Inspect and palpate gingiva

Use gloves to palpate.

■ *Color*	**EXPECTED:** Slightly stippled and pink. **UNEXPECTED:** Blue-black line about 1 mm from gum margin.
■ *Condition*	**EXPECTED:** Clearly defined, tight margin at each tooth. **UNEXPECTED:** Inflammation, swelling, bleeding, or lesions under dentures or on gingiva; induration, thickening, masses, or tenderness. Enlarged crevices between teeth and gum margins. Pockets containing debris at tooth margins.

Inspect tongue

■ *Size/symmetry*	**EXPECTED:** Midline. **UNEXPECTED:** Atrophied, deviation to one side.
■ *Color*	**EXPECTED:** Dull red.
■ *Dorsum surface* Have patient extend tongue and hold extended.	**EXPECTED:** Moist and glistening. *Anterior:* Smooth yet roughened surface with papillae and small fissures. *Posterior:* Smooth, slightly uneven or rugated surface with thinner mucosa than anterior. Possibly geographic.

TECHNIQUE	FINDINGS
	UNEXPECTED: Smooth, red, slick; hairy; swollen; coated; ulcerated; fasciculations; or limitation of movement.
■ *Ventral surface and floor of mouth* Have patient touch tip of tongue to palate behind upper incisors.	**EXPECTED:** Ventral surface pink and smooth with large veins between frenulum and fimbriated folds. Wharton ducts apparent on each side of frenulum. **UNEXPECTED:** Difficulty touching hard palate. Swelling, varicosities.
■ *Lateral borders* Wrap tongue with gauze and pull to each side. Scrape white or red margins to remove food particles.	**UNEXPECTED:** Leukoplakia or other fixed abnormality.

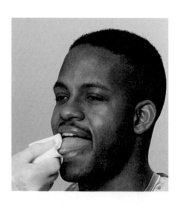

Palpate tongue and floor of mouth

	EXPECTED: Smooth and even. **UNEXPECTED:** Lumps, nodules, induration, ulcerations, or thickened white patches.

TECHNIQUE	FINDINGS

Inspect palate and uvula

Have patient tilt head back.

■ *Color and landmarks*

EXPECTED: Hard palate (whitish and dome shaped with transverse rugae) contiguous with pinker soft palate. Bony protuberance of hard palate at midline (torus palatinus).
UNEXPECTED: Nodule on palate, not at midline.

■ *Movement*
Ask patient to say "ah" while observing soft palate. (Depress tongue if necessary.)

EXPECTED: Soft palate rises symmetrically, with uvula remaining in midline.
UNEXPECTED: Failure of soft palate to rise bilaterally. Uvula deviation. Bifid uvula.

Inspect oropharynx

Depress tongue with tongue blade.

■ *Tonsils*

EXPECTED: Tonsils, if present, blend into pink color of pharynx. Possibly crypts in tonsils where cellular debris and food particles collect.
UNEXPECTED: Tonsils projecting beyond limits of tonsillar pillars. Tonsils red, enlarged, covered with exudate.

■ *Posterior wall of pharynx*

EXPECTED: Smooth, glistening, pink mucosa with some small, irregular spots of lymphatic tissue and small blood vessels.
UNEXPECTED: Red bulge adjacent to tonsil extending beyond midline. Yellowish mucoid film in pharynx. Grayish membrane.

TECHNIQUE	FINDINGS
Elicit gag reflex	**EXPECTED:** Bilateral response.
Touch posterior wall of pharynx on each side	**UNEXPECTED:** Unequal response or no response.

AIDS TO DIFFERENTIAL DIAGNOSIS

ABNORMALITY	DESCRIPTION
Acute otitis media	See table on p. 87.
Middle ear effusion (serous otitis media)	See table on p. 87.
Sinusitis	Fever, headache, local tenderness, pain, maxillary toothache, dull or opaque transillumination, colored nasal discharge, copious purulent nasal discharge.
Tonsillitis	Sore throat, referred pain to ears, dysphagia, fever, fetid breath, malaise. Tonsils are red and swollen. Tonsils covered with purulent exudate. May be studded with yellow follicles. Enlarged anterior cervical lymph nodes.
Peritonsillar abscess	Dysphagia, drooling, severe sore throat with pain radiating to ear, muffled voice, fever. Tonsil, tonsillar pillar, adjacent soft palate are red and swollen. Tonsil may appear pushed forward or backward, possibly displacing uvula.
Nasal polyps	Boggy mucosa, rounded, elongated, extending into nasal cavity.
Periodontal disease	Easily bleeding, swollen gums, enlarged crevices between teeth and gum margins.
Malocclusion	Teeth malpositioned, upper and lower molars not aligned, line of occlusion is incorrect.
Dental caries	Discolorations on crown.

Differentiating Between Otitis Externa, Acute Otitis Media, and Middle Ear Effusion

Signs and Symptoms	Otitis Externa	Acute Otitis Media	Middle Ear Effusion
Initial symptoms	Itching in ear canal	Fever, irritability, feeling of blockage, tugging at earlobe	Sticking or cracking sound on yawning or swallowing
Pain	Intense with movement of pinna or chewing	Deep-seated earache	Uncommon; feeling of fullness
Discharge	Watery, then purulent and thick, mixed with pus and epithelial cells; musty, foul smelling	Only if tympanic membrane ruptures; foul smelling	Uncommon
Hearing	Conductive loss caused by exudate and swelling of ear canal	Conductive loss as middle ear fills with pus	Conductive loss as middle ear fills with fluid
Inspection	Canal is red, edematous, tympanic membrane obscured	Tympanic membrane may be red, thickened, bulging; impaired movement	Tympanic membrane is retracted, yellowish; impaired mobility; visible air/fluid level and/or bubbles

PEDIATRIC VARIATIONS
EXAMINATION

TECHNIQUE	FINDINGS

Ears

Inspect tympanic membrane

In children, pull auricle downward and back.

EXPECTED: Tympanic membrane may be red from crying. If red from crying, it will be mobile.

Assess hearing

- *Evaluate response to auditory stimuli (bell, clapped hands, tissue paper)*

EXPECTED: For infants, see table below. Young children should turn toward sound consistently.

Nose and Sinuses

Evaluate patency of nares

With infant's mouth closed or with infant sucking on bottle or pacifier, occlude one naris and then the other. Observe respiratory pattern.

EXPECTED: Breathes easily; obligatory nose breathing until 2 to 3 months of age.

Sequences of Expected Hearing Response in Infants

Age	Response
Birth to 3 months	Startle reflex, crying, cessation of breathing or movement in response to sudden noise; quiets to parent's voice
4 to 6 months	Turns head toward source of sound but may not always recognize location of sound; responds to parent's voice; enjoys sound-producing toys
6 to 10 months	Responds to own name, telephone ringing, and person's voice, even if not loud; begins localizing sounds above and below, turns head 45 degrees toward sound
10 to 12 months	Recognizes and localizes source of sound; imitates simple words and sounds

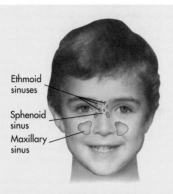

Ethmoid
sinuses

Sphenoid
sinus

Maxillary
sinus

TECHNIQUE	FINDINGS

Mouth

Inspect and palpate lips with mouth closed

EXPECTED: In infants aged 6 weeks to 6 months, sucking calluses, drooling.
UNEXPECTED: Drooling persistent after age 12 months.

Inspect teeth

■ *Color*

EXPECTED: 0 to 20 teeth until age 6 years. Permanent teeth start erupting around age 6 years.
UNEXPECTED: Natal teeth.

Inspect buccal mucosa

■ *Condition*

EXPECTED: In infants, nonadherent white patches (milk).
UNEXPECTED: In infants, adherent white patches.

Inspect and palpate gingiva

■ *Condition*

EXPECTED: In infants, pearl-like retention cysts.

AIDS TO DIFFERENTIAL DIAGNOSIS

ABNORMALITY	DESCRIPTION
Epiglottitis	High fever, croupy cough, sore throat, drooling, difficulty breathing.

SAMPLE DOCUMENTATION

Subjective. A 55-year-old man with concerns about hearing loss for the past few months, particularly with high-pitched tones. Has difficulty hearing on phone and in conversations when multiple people are talking. Hears "noise" in both ears when trying to go to sleep at night. No ear pain or discharge. No nasal discharge or sinus pain. No mouth lesions or masses; no recent dental problems; no sore throat.

Objective. *Ears:* Auricles in alignment. Canals totally obstructed by cerumen bilaterally. After irrigation, tympanic membranes are pearly gray, noninjected, intact, with bony landmarks and light reflex visualized bilaterally. No evidence of fluid or retraction. Conversational hearing appropriate. Able to hear whispered voice. Weber—lateralizes equally to both ears, Rinne—air conduction greater than bone conduction bilaterally (30 seconds/15 seconds). *Nose:* No discharge or polyps, mucosa pink and moist, septum midline, patent bilaterally. No edema over frontal or maxillary sinuses. No sinus tenderness to palpation. Correctly identifies mint, banana, ammonia odors. *Mouth:* Buccal mucosa pink and moist without lesions. Twenty-six teeth present in various states of repair. Lower second molars (18, 30) absent bilaterally. Gingiva pink and firm. Tongue midline with no tremors or fasciculation. Pharynx clear without erythema; tonsils 1+ without exudates. Uvula rises evenly, and gag reflex is intact. No hoarseness. Patient identifies tastes of salt and sugar.

9

mosby.com/MERLIN/Seidel

Chest and Lungs

EQUIPMENT

- Drape
- Skin-marking pencil
- Ruler and tape measure
- Stethoscope with bell and diaphragm

EXAMINATION

Have patient sit, disrobed to waist.

TECHNIQUE	FINDINGS
Inspect front and back of chest	
See thoracic landmarks.	
■ *Size/shape/symmetry*	
■ *Landmarks*	**EXPECTED:** Supernumerary nipples possible (but could be clue to other congenital abnormalities).

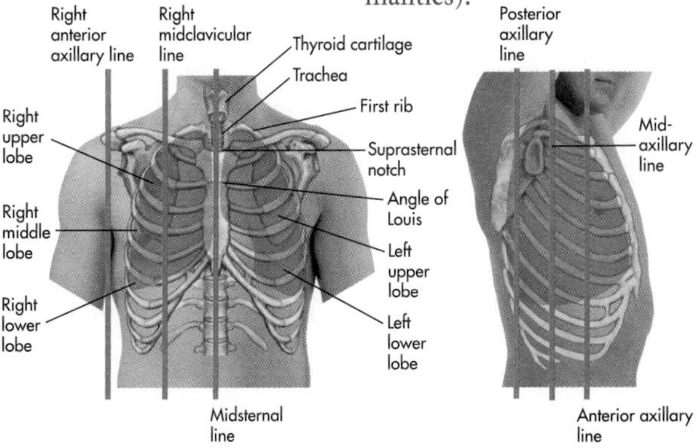

Right anterior axillary line
Right midclavicular line
Thyroid cartilage
Trachea
First rib
Right upper lobe
Suprasternal notch
Angle of Louis
Right middle lobe
Left upper lobe
Right lower lobe
Left lower lobe
Midsternal line
Posterior axillary line
Mid-axillary line
Anterior axillary line

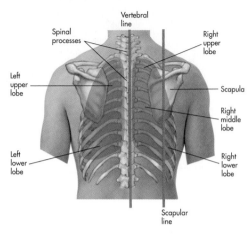

TECHNIQUE	FINDINGS
■ *Compare anteroposterior diameter with transverse diameter*	**EXPECTED:** Ribs prominent, clavicles prominent superiorly, sternum usually flat and free of abundance of overlying tissue. Chest somewhat asymmetric. Anteroposterior diameter often one half of transverse diameter. **UNEXPECTED:** Barrel chest, posterior or lateral deviation, pigeon chest, or funnel chest.
■ *Assess nails, lips, nares*	**UNEXPECTED:** Clubbed fingernails, pursed lips, flared alae nasi.
■ *Color* Assess skin, lips, nails.	**UNEXPECTED:** Superficial venous patterns. Cyanosis or pallor of lips or nails.
■ *Breath*	**UNEXPECTED:** Malodorous.

Evaluate respirations

■ *Rhythm or pattern and rate*
See patterns of respiration in figure on p. 93.

EXPECTED: Breathing easy, regular, without distress. Pattern even. Rate 12 to 20 respirations per minute. Ratio of respirations to heartbeats about 1:4.

Normal	Regular and comfortable at a rate of 12-20 per minute	Air trapping	Increasing difficulty in getting breath out
Bradypnea	Slower than 12 breaths per minute	Cheyne-Stokes	Varying periods of increasing depth interspersed with apnea
Tachypnea	Faster than 20 breaths per minute	Kussmaul	Rapid, deep, labored
Hyperventilation (hyperpnea)	Faster than 20 breaths per minute, deep breathing	Biot	Irregularly interspersed periods of apnea in a disorganized sequence of breaths
Sighing	Frequently interspersed deeper breath	Ataxic	Significant disorganization with irregular and varying depths of respiration

TECHNIQUE	FINDINGS
	UNEXPECTED: Dyspnea, orthopnea, paroxysmal nocturnal dyspnea, platypnea, tachypnea, hypopnea. Use of accessory muscles, retractions.
■ *Inspiration/expiration ratio*	**UNEXPECTED:** Air trapping, prolonged expiration.

Inspect chest movement with breathing

■ *Symmetry*	**EXPECTED:** Chest expansion bilaterally symmetric.
	UNEXPECTED: Asymmetry. Unilateral or bilateral bulging. Bulging on expiration.

Listen to respiration sounds audible without stethoscope

	EXPECTED: Generally bronchovesicular.

TECHNIQUE	FINDINGS
	UNEXPECTED: Crepitus, stridor, wheezes.

Palpate thoracic muscles and skeleton

■ *Symmetry/condition*

EXPECTED: Bilateral symmetry. Some elasticity of rib cage, but sternum and xiphoid relatively inflexible and thoracic spine rigid.

UNEXPECTED: Pulsations, tenderness, bulges, depressions, unusual movement, unusual positions.

■ *Thoracic expansion*
Stand behind patient. Place palms in light contact with posterolateral surfaces and thumbs along spinal processes at tenth rib, as shown in figure at right. Watch thumb divergence during quiet and deep breathing. Face patient; place thumbs along costal margin and xiphoid process with palms touching anterolateral chest. Watch thumb divergence during quiet and deep breathing.

EXPECTED: Symmetric expansion.

UNEXPECTED: Asymmetric expansion.

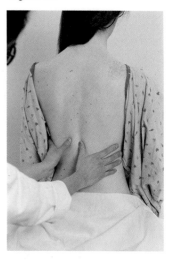

■ *Sensations*

EXPECTED: Nontender sensations.

UNEXPECTED: Crepitus or grating vibration.

TECHNIQUE	FINDINGS
■ *Tactile fremitus* Ask patient to recite numbers or words while systematically palpating chest with palmar surfaces of fingers or ulnar aspect of clenched fist, using firm, light touch. Assess each area, front to back, side to side, lung apices. Compare sides.	**EXPECTED:** Great variability. **UNEXPECTED:** Decreased or absent fremitus; increased fremitus (coarser, rougher); or gentle, more tremulous fremitus. Variation between similar positions on right and left thorax.
Note position of trachea Using index finger or thumbs, palpate gently from suprasternal notch along upper edges of each clavicle and in spaces above, to inner borders of sternocleidomastoid muscles.	**EXPECTED:** Spaces equal side to side. Trachea midline directly above suprasternal notch. Possible slight deviation to right. **UNEXPECTED:** Significant deviation or tug. Pulsations.

Perform direct or indirect percussion on chest

Percuss directly or indirectly, as shown in figures below. Compare all areas bilaterally, following a sequence such as shown in top figures on p. 96.

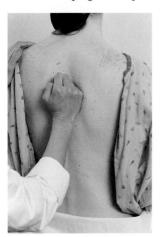
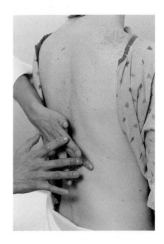

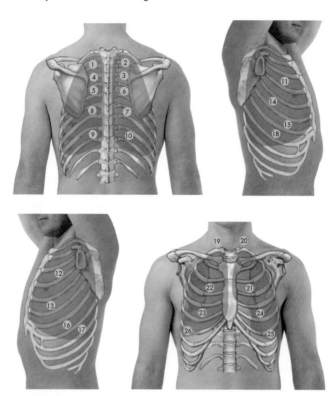

Percussion Tones Heard Over the Chest

Type of Tone	Intensity	Pitch	Duration	Quality
Resonant	Loud	Low	Long	Hollow
Flat	Soft	High	Short	Extremely dull
Dull	Medium	Medium-high	Medium	Thudlike
Tympanic	Loud	High	Medium	Drumlike
Hyperresonant*	Very loud	Very low	Longer	Booming

From Thompson et al, 1997.
*Hyperresonance is unexpected in adults. It represents air trapping, which occurs in obstructive lung diseases.

TECHNIQUE	FINDINGS

See table on p. 96 for common tones, intensity, pitch, duration, quality.

- *Thorax*
Have patient sit with head bent and arms folded in front while percussing posterior thorax, then with arms raised overhead while percussing lateral and anterior chest. Percuss at 4- to 5-cm intervals over intercostal spaces, moving superior to inferior, medial to lateral.

EXPECTED: Resonance over all areas of lungs, dull over heart and liver, spleen, areas of thorax.
UNEXPECTED: Hyperresonance, dullness, or flatness.

- *Diaphragmatic excursion*
Ask patient to breathe deeply and hold breath. Percuss along scapular line on one side until tone changes from resonant to dull. Mark skin. Allow patient to breathe normally, then repeat on other side. Have patient take several breaths, then exhale as much as possible and hold. On each side, percuss up from mark to change from dull to resonant. Tell patient to resume breathing comfortably. Measure excursion distance.

EXPECTED: 3 to 5 cm (higher on right than left).
UNEXPECTED: Limited descent.

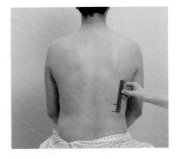

TECHNIQUE	FINDINGS

Auscultate chest with stethoscope diaphragm, apex to base

- *Intensity, pitch, duration, and quality of breath sounds*
  Have patient breathe slowly and deeply through mouth. Follow set auscultation sequence, holding stethoscope as shown in figure at right. Ask patient to sit upright (1) with head bent and arms folded in front while auscultating posterior thorax, (2) with arms raised overhead while auscultating lateral chest, (3) with arms down and shoulders back while auscultating anterior chest.

EXPECTED: See expected breath sounds in table below.
UNEXPECTED: Amphoric or cavernous breathing. Sounds difficult to hear or absent. Crackles, rhonchi, wheezes, or pleural friction rub, as described in box on p. 99.

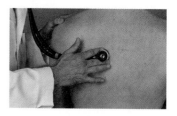

Characteristics of Expected Breath Sounds

Sound	Characteristics	Findings
Vesicular	Heard over most of lung fields; low pitch; soft and short expirations; will be accentuated in a thin person or a child and diminished in overweight or very muscular patient	
Bronchovesicular	Heard over main bronchus area and over upper right posterior lung field; medium pitch; expiration equals inspiration	
Bronchial tracheal (tubular)	Heard only over trachea; high pitch; loud and long expirations, often somewhat longer than inspiration	

Modified from Thompson et al, 1997.

TECHNIQUE   FINDINGS

Listen during inspiration and
expiration. Auscultate downward from apex to base at intervals of several centimeters,
making side-to-side compar-
isons.

Adventitious Breath Sounds

Fine crackles: High-pitched, discrete, discontinuous crackling
sounds heard during end of inspiration; not cleared by cough

Medium crackles: Lower, more
moist sound heard during mid-
stage of inspiration; not
cleared by cough

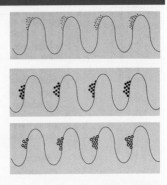

Coarse crackles: Loud, bubbly
noise heard during inspiration;
not cleared by cough

Rhonchi (sonorous wheeze):
Loud, low, coarse sounds, like
a snore, most often heard con-
tinuously during inspiration or
expiration; coughing may clear
sound (usually means mucus
accumulation in trachea or
large bronchi)

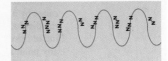

Wheeze (sibilant wheeze):
Musical noise sounding like a
squeak; most often heard con-
tinuously during inspiration or
expiration; usually louder during expiration

Pleural friction rub: Dry rubbing
or grating sound, usually
caused by inflammation of
pleural surfaces; heard during
inspiration or expiration; loud-
est over lower lateral anterior
surface

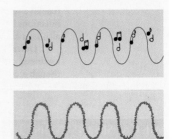

Modified from Thompson et al, 1997.

TECHNIQUE	FINDINGS
■ *Vocal resonance* Ask patient to recite numbers or words.	**EXPECTED:** Muffled and indistinct sounds. **UNEXPECTED:** Bronchophony, whispered pectoriloquy, or egophony.

AIDS TO DIFFERENTIAL DIAGNOSIS

ABNORMALITY	DESCRIPTION
Lung cancer	Cough, wheezing, emphysema, atelectasis, pneumonitis, hemoptysis. Possible sputum.
Infections	Sputum production (see table below).
Cough-producing conditions	See box on p. 101.
Asthma	Cough, wheezing, respiratory distress, tachypnea, pallor to cyanosis; possible decreased breath sounds; possibly allergy or exercise induced.
Chronic obstructive pulmonary disease	Barrel chest, hyperresonance to percussion, sputum production, cough, prolonged expiration, amphoric breathing.

Assessing Sputum

Cause	Possible Sputum Characteristics
Bacterial infection	Yellow, green, rust-colored (blood mixed with yellow sputum), clear, or transparent; purulent; blood streaked; mucoid, viscid
Viral infection	Mucoid, viscid; blood streaked (not common)
Chronic infectious disease	All of the above; particularly abundant in early morning; slight, intermittent blood streaking; occasionally large amounts of blood
Carcinoma	Slight, persistent blood streaking
Infarction	Blood clotted; large amounts of blood
Tuberculous cavity	Large amounts of blood

Assessing Cough

Coughs are common symptoms of a respiratory problem. They are usually preceded by a deep inspiration; this is followed by closure of the glottis, relaxation of the diaphragm, and then a sudden, spasmodic expiration, forcing a sudden opening of the glottis. Causes may be related to localized or more general insults at any point in the respiratory tract. Coughs may be voluntary, but they are usually reflexive responses to an irritant such as a foreign body (microscopic or larger), an infectious agent, or a mass of any sort compressing the respiratory tree. They may also be a clue to an anxiety state.

Describe a cough according to its moisture, frequency, regularity, pitch and loudness, quality. The type of cough may offer some clue to the cause. Although a cough may not have a serious cause, it should not be ignored.

Dry or moist. A moist cough may be caused by infection and can be accompanied by sputum production. A dry cough can have a variety of causes (e.g., cardiac problems, allergies, or AIDS), which may be indicated by the quality of its sound.

Onset. Acute onset, particularly with fever, suggests infection; in the absence of fever, a foreign body or inhaled irritants are additional possible causes.

Frequency of occurrence. Note whether the cough is seldom or often present. Infrequent cough may result from allergens or environmental insults.

Regularity. A regular, paroxysmal cough is heard in pertussis. Irregularly occurring cough may have a variety of causes, such as smoking, early congestive heart failure, an inspired foreign body or irritant, or a tumor within or compressing the bronchial tree.

Pitch and loudness. A cough may be loud and high pitched or quiet and relatively low pitched.

Postural influences. A cough may occur soon after a person has reclined or assumed an erect position (e.g., with a nasal drip or pooling of secretions in the upper airway).

Quality. A dry cough may sound brassy if it is caused by compression of the respiratory tree (as by a tumor) or hoarse if it is caused by croup. Pertussis produces an inspiratory "whoop" at the end of a paroxysm of coughing.

PEDIATRIC VARIATIONS
EXAMINATION

TECHNIQUE	FINDINGS

Inspect front and back of chest

- *Compare anteroposterior diameter with transverse diameter*

EXPECTED: Infant's chest is expected to measure 2 to 3 cm less than head circumference.

Evaluate respirations

- *Rhythm or pattern and rate*

EXPECTED:

AGE	RESPIRATIONS PER MINUTE
Newborn	30-80
1 year	20-40
3 years	20-30
6 years	16-22
10 years	16-20
17 years	12-20

Perform direct or indirect percussion on chest

- *Thorax*

EXPECTED: Hyperresonance may be heard in children.

Auscultate chest with stethoscope diaphragm, apex to base

- *Intensity, pitch, duration, and quality of breath sounds*

EXPECTED: In infants and children, expect transmitted breath sounds throughout chest. Vesicular sound will be accentuated in a child. Absent or diminished breath sounds are harder to detect.

Subjective. A 45-year-old woman complaining of cough and fever for 4 days. Cough is nonproductive, persistent, and worse when she lies down. She feels ill and short of breath. Her chest feels "heavy." Fever up to 38.3° C (101° F). Taking acetaminophen and over-the-counter cough syrup without relief.

Objective. Minimal increase in anteroposterior diameter of chest, without kyphosis or other defect. Trachea in midline without tug. Thoracic expansion symmetric. Respirations 32 per minute and somewhat labored; no retractions or stridor. No friction rubs or tenderness over ribs or other bony prominences. Over posterior left base, diminished tactile fremitus, dull percussion note; and on auscultation, crackles that do not clear with cough, diminished breath sounds. Remaining lung fields are clear and free of adventitious sounds, with resonant percussion tones. Diaphragmatic excursion 3 cm bilaterally.

Clinical and Reference Notes

10

Heart

EQUIPMENT

- Tangential light source
- Skin-marking pencil
- Stethoscope with bell and diaphragm
- Centimeter ruler

EXAMINATION

TECHNIQUE	FINDINGS

Heart

Inspect precordium

Have patient supine, and keep light source tangential.

- *Apical impulse*

EXPECTED: Visible about mid-clavicular line in fifth left intercostal space. Sometimes visible only with patient sitting.

UNEXPECTED: Visible in more than one intercostal space; exaggerated lifts or heaves.

TECHNIQUE	FINDINGS

Palpate precordium

■ *Apical impulse*
Have patient supine. With hands *warm,* gently feel precordium, using proximal halves of fingers held together or whole hand. As shown in figure at right, methodically move from apex to left sternal border, base, right sternal border, epigastrium, axillae. Locate sensation in terms of its intercostal space and relationship to midsternal, midclavicular, axillary lines.

EXPECTED: Gentle, brief impulse, palpable within radius of 1 cm or less, although often not felt.
UNEXPECTED: Heave or lift, loss of thrust, displacement to right or left; thrill.

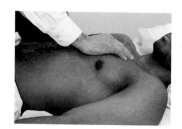

Percuss precordium (optional)

Begin by tapping at anterior axillary line, moving medially along intercostal spaces toward sternal borders until tone changes from resonance to dullness. Mark skin with pencil.

EXPECTED: No change in tone before right sternal border; on left, loss of resonance generally close to point of maximal impulse at fifth intercostal space. Loss of resonance may outline left border of heart at second to fifth intercostal spaces.

TECHNIQUE	FINDINGS

Auscultate in five auscultatory areas

Make certain patient is warm and relaxed. Isolate each sound and each pause in cycle, and then inch along with stethoscope. Approach each of the five precordial areas shown in figure below systematically, base to apex or apex to base, using each position shown in figures at right. Use diaphragm of stethoscope first, with firm pressure, then bell, with light pressure.

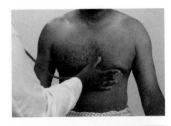

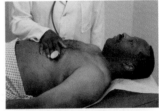

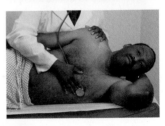

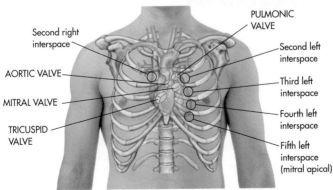

PULMONIC VALVE

Second right interspace

AORTIC VALVE

MITRAL VALVE

TRICUSPID VALVE

Second left interspace

Third left interspace

Fourth left interspace

Fifth left interspace (mitral apical)

TECHNIQUE	FINDINGS
■ *Rate and rhythm* Assess overall rate and rhythm.	**EXPECTED:** Rate 60 to 90 beats per minute, regular rhythm. **UNEXPECTED:** Bradycardia, tachycardia, arrhythmia.
■ S_1 Ask patient to breathe comfortably, then hold breath in expiration. Listen for S_1 (best heard toward apex) while palpating carotid pulse. Note intensity, variations, effect of respiration, splitting. Concentrate on systole, then diastole.	**EXPECTED:** S_1 usually heard as one sound and coincides with rise of carotid pulse. See table below and figure on p. 109. **UNEXPECTED:** Extra sounds or murmurs.
■ S_2 Ask patient to breathe comfortably as you listen for S_2 (best heard in aortic and pulmonic areas) to become two components during inspiration. Ask patient to inhale and hold breath.	**EXPECTED:** S_2 to become two components during inspiration. S_2 to become an apparent single sound as breath exhaled. See table below and figure on p. 109.

Heart Sounds According to Auscultatory Area

	Aortic	Pulmonic	Second Pulmonic	Mitral	Tricuspid
Pitch	$S_1 < S_2$	$S_1 < S_2$	$S_1 < S_2$	$S_1 < S_2$	$S_1 < S_2$
Loudness	$S_1 < S_2$	$S_1 < S_2$	$S_1 < S_2$*	$S_1 > S_2$†	$S_1 > S_2$
Duration	$S_1 > S_2$	$S_1 > S_2$	$S_1 > S_2$	$S_1 > S_2$	$S_1 > S_2$
S_2 split	>Inhale	>Inhale	>Inhale	>Inhale‡	>Inhale
	<Exhale	<Exhale	<Exhale	<Exhale	<Exhale
A_2	Loudest	Loud	Decreased		
P_2	Decreased	Louder	Loudest		

*S_1 is relatively louder in second pulmonic area than in aortic area.
†S_1 may be louder in mitral area than in tricuspid area.
‡S_2 split may not be audible in mitral area if P_2 is inaudible.

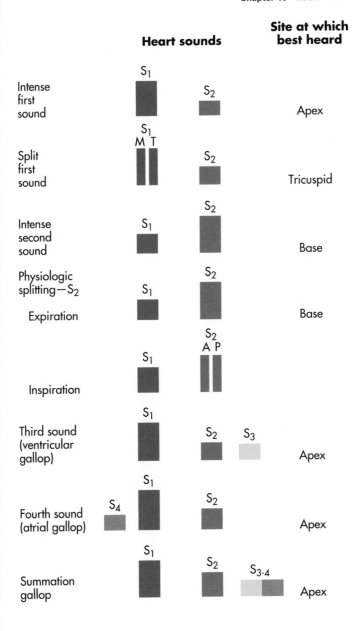

TECHNIQUE	FINDINGS
■ *Splitting*	**EXPECTED:** S_2 splitting—greatest at peak of inspiration—varying from easily heard to nondetectable.
■ *S_3 and S_4* If needed, ask patient to raise a leg to increase venous return or to grip your hand vigorously and repeatedly to increase venous return.	**EXPECTED:** Both S_3 and S_4 quiet and difficult to hear. S_3 has rhythm of Ken-tuc-ky; S_4, Tenn-es-see. **UNEXPECTED:** Increased intensity (and ease of hearing) of either.
■ *Extra heart sounds*	**UNEXPECTED:** Extra heart sounds—snaps, clicks, friction rubs, murmurs. See table on p. 111 and figure on p. 109.

Assess characteristics of murmurs

■ *Timing and duration, pitch, intensity, pattern, quality, location, radiation, respiratory phase variations*

AIDS TO DIFFERENTIAL DIAGNOSIS

ABNORMALITY	DESCRIPTION
Chest pain	See table on p. 112.
Left ventricular hypertrophy	Vigorous sustained lift palpable during ventricular systole, sometimes over broader area than usual (by 2 cm or more). Displacement of apical impulse can be well lateral of midclavicular line and downward.

Extra Heart Sounds

Sound	Detection	Description
Increased S_3	Bell at apex; patient left lateral recumbent	Early diastole, low pitch
Increased S_4	Bell apex; patient supine or semilateral	Late diastole or early systole, low pitch
Gallops	Bell at apex; patient supine or left lateral recumbent	Presystole, intense, easily heard
Mitral valve opening snap	Diaphragm medial to apex, may radiate to base; any position, second left intercostal	Early diastole briefly, before S_3; high pitch, sharp snap or click; not affected by respiration; easily confused with S_2
Ejection clicks	Diaphragm; patient sitting or supine	
Aortic valve	Apex, base in second right intercostal space	Early systole, intense, high pitch; radiates, not affected by respirations
Pulmonary valve	Second left intercostal space at sternal border	Early systole, less intense than aortic click; intensifies on expiration, decreases on inspiration
Pericardial friction rub	Widely heard, sound clearest toward apex	May occupy all of systole and diastole; intense, grating, machinelike; may have three components and obliterate heart sounds; if only one or two components, may sound like murmur

Chest Pain

Type of Chest Pain	Characteristics
Anginal	Substernal; provoked by effort, emotion, eating; relieved by rest and/or nitroglycerin
Pleural	Precipitated by breathing or coughing; usually described as sharp
Esophageal	Burning, substernal, occasional radiation to shoulder; nocturnal occurrence, usually when lying flat; relief with food, antacids, sometimes nitroglycerin
From a peptic ulcer	Almost always infradiaphragmatic and epigastric; nocturnal occurrence and daytime attacks relieved by food; unrelated to activity
Biliary	Usually under right scapula, prolonged in duration; will trigger angina more often than mimic it
From arthritis/bursitis	Usually of hours-long duration; local tenderness and/or pain with movement
Cervical	Associated with injury; provoked by activity, persists after activity; painful on palpation and/or movement
Musculoskeletal (chest)	Intensified or provoked by movement, particularly twisting or costochondral bending; long lasting; often associated with local tenderness
Psychoneurotic	Associated with or occurring after anxiety; poorly described, located in intramammary region

Data from Samiy et al, 1987; Harvey et al, 1988.

ABNORMALITY	DESCRIPTION
Right ventricular hypertrophy	Lift along left sternal border in third and fourth left intercostal spaces accompanied by occasional systolic retraction at apex. Left ventricle displaced and turned posteriorly by enlarged right ventricle.
Congestive heart failure	Congestion in pulmonary or systemic circulation. Can be predominantly left- or right-sided and can develop gradually or suddenly with acute pulmonary edema.
Cor pulmonale	Left parasternal systolic lift and loud S_2 in pulmonic region.
Myocardial infarction	Deep substernal or visceral pain, often radiating to jaw, neck, left arm (although discomfort is sometimes mild); dysrhythmias; S_4 often present. Heart sounds distant, with soft, systolic, blowing murmur; pulse possibly thready; varied blood pressure (although hypertension usual in early phases).
Myocarditis	*Initial:* Fatigue, dyspnea, fever, palpitations. *Later:* Cardiac enlargement, murmur, gallop rhythms, tachycardia, dysrhythmias, pulsus alternans.
Conduction disturbances	Transient weakness, fainting spells, or strokelike episodes.
Atherosclerotic heart disease	May cause myocardial insufficiency, angina pectoris, dysrhythmias, congestive heart failure.

ABNORMALITY	DESCRIPTION
Angina	Substernal pain or intense pressure radiating at times to neck, jaws, arms, particularly left arm. Often accompanied by shortness of breath, fatigue, diaphoresis, faintness, syncope. Cessation of activity may relieve pain.

PEDIATRIC VARIATIONS

EXAMINATION

TECHNIQUE	FINDINGS
Assess characteristics of murmurs	
■ *Timing and duration, intensity, pattern, quality, location, radiation, respiratory phase variations*	In children it is necessary to distinguish innocent murmurs from organic murmurs caused by congenital defect or rheumatic fever.

AIDS TO DIFFERENTIAL DIAGNOSIS

ABNORMALITY	DESCRIPTION
Chest pain	Unlike in adults, chest pain in children and adolescents is seldom caused by a cardiac problem. It is very often difficult to find a cause, but trauma and exercise-induced asthma and use of cocaine, even in a somewhat younger child, as in the adolescent and adult, should be among the considerations.
Congenital defects Tetralogy of Fallot	Parasternal heave and precordial prominence. Cyanosis. Systolic ejection murmur heard over third intercostal space, sometimes radiating to left side of neck. Single S_2.

ABNORMALITY	DESCRIPTION
Ventricular septal defect	Arterial pulse small, and jugular venous pulse unaffected. Regurgitation occurs through septal defect, resulting in holosystolic murmur that is frequently loud, coarse, high-pitched, best heard along left sternal border in third to fifth intercostal spaces. Distinct lift often discernible along left sternal border and apical area. Does not radiate to neck.
Patent ductus arteriosus	Neck vessels dilated and pulsate, and pulse pressure wide. Harsh, loud, continuous murmur with machinelike quality, heard at first to third intercostal spaces and lower sternal border. Murmur usually unaltered by postural change.
Atrial septal defect	Systolic ejection murmur—best heard over pulmonic area—that is diamond shaped, often loud, high in pitch, and harsh. May be accompanied by brief, rumbling, early diastolic murmur. Does not usually radiate beyond precordium. Systolic thrill may be felt over area of murmur along with palpable parasternal thrust. S_2 may be split fairly widely. Particularly significant with palpable thrust and occasional radiation through to back.
Dextrocardia and situs inversus	Altered clinical manifestations of disease (e.g., substernal pressure of myocardial ischemia) may be felt to right of precordium and may more often radiate to right arm.

Heart. No visible pulsations over precordium. Point of maximal impulse (PMI) palpable at the fifth ICS in the MCL, 1 cm in diameter. No lifts, heaves, or thrills felt on palpation. S_1 is crisp. Split S_2 increases with inspiration. No audible S_3, S_4, murmur, click, or rub.

11

Blood Vessels

EQUIPMENT

- Tangential light source
- Stethoscope with bell and diaphragm
- Sphygmomanometer
- Centimeter ruler

EXAMINATION

TECHNIQUE   FINDINGS

Peripheral Arteries

Palpate arterial pulses in neck and extremities

Palpate carotid, brachial, radial, femoral, popliteal, dorsalis pedis, and posterior tibial arteries, using distal pads
of second and third fingers,
as shown in figures on p. 118.

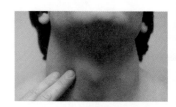

Carotid.

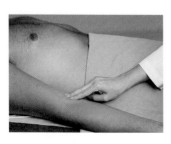

Brachial.

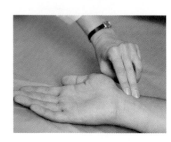

Radial.

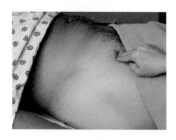

Femoral.

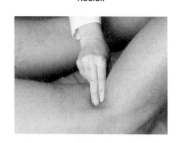

Popliteal.

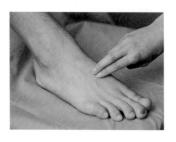

Dorsalis pedis.

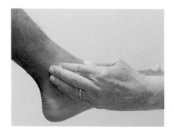

Posterior tibial.

TECHNIQUE	FINDINGS

- *Characteristics*
Compare characteristics bilaterally, as well as between
upper and lower extremities.

EXPECTED: Femoral pulse as
strong as or stronger than radial
pulse.
UNEXPECTED: Femoral pulse
weaker than radial pulse or absent. Alternating pulse (pulsus
alternans), pulsus bisferiens,
bigeminal pulse (pulsus bigemi-
nus), bounding pulse, labile
pulse, paradoxic pulse (pulsus
paradoxus), pulsus differens,
tachycardia, trigeminal pulse
(pulsus trigeminus), or water-
hammer pulse (Corrigan pulse).

- *Rate*

EXPECTED: 60 to 90 beats per
minute.
UNEXPECTED: Rate different
from that observed during cardiac examination.

- *Rhythm*

EXPECTED: Regular.
UNEXPECTED: Irregular, either
in a pattern or patternless.

- *Contour*

EXPECTED: Smooth, rounded,
or dome shaped.

- *Amplitude*

UNEXPECTED: Bounding, full,
diminished, or absent.
Describe on scale of 0 to 4:
0 = Absent, not palpable
1 = Diminished
2 = Expected
3 = Full, increased
4 = Bounding

TECHNIQUE	FINDINGS

Auscultate temporal, carotid, and subclavian arteries; abdominal aorta; and renal, iliac, and femoral arteries for bruits

You may at times need to ask patient to hold breath for a few heartbeats. Auscultate with bell of stethoscope.

UNEXPECTED: Transmitted murmurs, bruits.

Assess for arterial occlusion and insufficiency

■ *Site*
Assess for pain distal to possible occlusion.

UNEXPECTED: Dull ache accompanied by fatigue and often crampiness; possible constant or excruciating pain. Weak, thready, or absent pulses; systolic bruits over arteries; loss of body warmth; localized pallor or cyanosis; delay in venous filling; or thin, atrophied skin, muscle atrophy, and loss of hair.

■ *Degree of occlusion*
Ask patient to lie supine. Elevate extremity, note degree of blanching, then ask patient to sit on edge of table or bed to lower extremity. Note time for maximal return of color when extremity is lowered.

EXPECTED: Slight pallor on elevation and return to full color as soon as leg becomes dependent.
UNEXPECTED: Delay of more than 2 seconds.

Measure blood pressure

Measure in both arms at least once. Patient's arm should be slightly flexed and comfortably supported on table, pillow, or your hand.

EXPECTED: 100 to 140 mm Hg systolic and 60 to 90 mm Hg second diastolic, with pulse pressure of 30 to 40 mm Hg (sometimes to 50 mm Hg). Reading between arms may vary by as much as 10 mm Hg; usually higher in right arm.
UNEXPECTED: Hypertension (see table on p. 121).

**Classification of Blood Pressure for Adults Aged
18 Years and Older***

Category	Systolic (mm Hg)		Diastolic (mm Hg)
Optimal†	<120	and	<80
Normal	<130	and	<85
High-normal	130-139	or	85-89
Hypertension‡			
Stage 1	140-159	or	90-99
Stage 2	160-179	or	100-109
Stage 3	≥180	or	≥110

From NIH Publication No. 48-4080, November 1997.
*Not taking antihypertensive drugs and not acutely ill. When systolic and diastolic blood pressures fall into different categories, the higher category should be selected to classify the individual's blood pressure status. For example, 160/92 mm Hg should be classified as stage 2 hypertension, and 124/120 mm Hg should be classified as stage 3 hypertension. Isolated systolic hypertension is defined as systolic blood pressure of 140 mm Hg or greater and diastolic blood pressure below 90 mm Hg and staged appropriately (e.g., 170/82 mm Hg is defined as stage 2 isolated systolic hypertension). In addition to classifying stages of hypertension on the basis of average blood pressure levels, clinicians should specify presence or absence of target organ disease and additional risk factors. Specificity is important for risk classification and treatment.
†Optimal blood pressure with respect to cardiovascular risk is below 120/80 mm Hg. However, unusually low readings should be evaluated for clinical significance.
‡Based on the average of two or more readings taken at each of two or more visits after an initial screening.

TECHNIQUE	FINDINGS

Peripheral Veins

Assess jugular venous pressure

Ask patient to recline at 45-degree angle. With tangential light, observe both jugular veins. As shown in figure at right, use a centimeter ruler to measure vertical distance between midaxillary line and highest level of jugular vein distention.

EXPECTED: Pressure 9 cm H$_2$O or less, bilaterally symmetric.
UNEXPECTED: Abnormal distention or distention on one side.

Assess for venous obstruction and insufficiency

Inspect extremities, with patient both standing and supine.

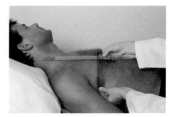

TECHNIQUE	FINDINGS
■ *Affected area*	**UNEXPECTED:** Constant pain with swelling and tenderness over muscles, engorgement of superficial veins, cyanosis.
■ *Thrombosis* Flex patient's knee slightly with one hand, and with other, dorsiflex foot to test for Homans sign.	**UNEXPECTED:** Redness, thickening, tenderness along superficial vein. Calf pain with test for Homans sign.
■ *Edema* Press index finger over bony prominence of tibia or medial malleolus for several seconds.	**UNEXPECTED:** Orthostatic (pitting) edema; thickening and ulceration of skin possible. Grade edema from 1+ to 4+ as follows: 1+ = Slight pitting, no visible distortion, disappears rapidly 2+ = Deeper than 1+ and disappears in 10 to 15 seconds 3+ = Noticeably deep and may last more than 1 minute, with dependent extremity full and swollen 4+ = Very deep and lasts 2 to 5 minutes, with grossly distorted dependent extremity
■ *Varicose veins* If suspected, have patient stand on toes 10 times in succession.	**EXPECTED:** Pressure from toe standing disappears in seconds. **UNEXPECTED:** Veins dilated and swollen; often tortuous when extremities are dependent and pressure does not quickly disappear.
If varicose veins are present, assess venous incompetence with Trendelenburg test: Ask patient to lie supine, lift leg above heart level until veins empty, then quickly lower leg.	**UNEXPECTED:** Rapid filling of veins.

TECHNIQUE	FINDINGS
Evaluate patency of deep veins with Perthes test: Ask patient to lie supine. Elevate extremity, and occlude subcutaneous veins with tourniquet just above knee. Then ask patient to walk.	**UNEXPECTED:** Superficial veins fail to empty.
Evaluate direction of blood flow and presence of compensatory circulation: Put affected limb in dependent position, then empty or strip vein. Release pressure of one finger nearest heart to assess blood flow; if necessary, repeat and release pressure of other finger.	**UNEXPECTED:** Stripped vessel fills before pressure is released, or blood refills entire vein when pressure is released.

AIDS TO DIFFERENTIAL DIAGNOSIS

ABNORMALITY	DESCRIPTION
Arterial aneurysm	Pulsatile dilatation along course of an artery—most commonly in the aorta, although intracranial, abdominal, renal, femoral, and popliteal arteries are also affected. Thrill or bruit sometimes evident over aneurysm.
Venous thrombosis	Clinical findings in superficial vein include redness, thickening, tenderness along involved segment. Deep vein thrombosis in femoral and pelvic circulations may be asymptomatic, but suggestive signs and symptoms include tenderness along iliac vessels and femoral canal, in popliteal space, and over deep calf veins, as well as slight swelling, minimal ankle edema, low-grade fever, and tachycardia.

ABNORMALITY	DESCRIPTION
Raynaud disease	Intermittent skin pallor followed by cyanosis, bilateral and lasting from minutes to hours. Skin over digits eventually appears smooth, shiny, tight; ulcers may appear on tips of digits.

PEDIATRIC VARIATIONS

TECHNIQUE	FINDINGS
Palpate arterial pulses in distal extremities	
■ *Rate*	**EXPECTED:**

AGE	BEATS PER MINUTE
Newborn	120-170
1 year	80-160
3 years	80-120
6 years	75-115
10 years	70-110

TECHNIQUE	FINDINGS
Auscultate arteries for bruits	**EXPECTED:** In children it is not unusual to hear a venous hum over internal jugular veins. There is usually no pathologic significance.
Measure blood pressure	
When measuring an infant's blood pressure, use flush technique if needed.	**EXPECTED:** Calculation of systolic blood pressure for children older than 1 year can be estimated with following formula: $80 + (2 \times$ Child's age in years) Example: Calculation of expected systolic blood pressure of 5-year-old child: $80 + (2 \times 5) = 90$ Although this calculation gives a figure below the expected mean, it is still considered within normal limits for a 5-year-old child. **UNEXPECTED:** Hypertension (see tables on pp. 126-129).

AIDS TO DIFFERENTIAL DIAGNOSIS

ABNORMALITY	DESCRIPTION
Coarctation of the aorta	Delay and/or palpable diminution in amplitude (not necessarily an absence) of femoral pulse when radial and femoral pulses are palpated simultaneously. Findings are same on right and left sides. Blood pressure in arms will be distinctly, even dramatically, higher than in legs. Possible systolic murmur audible over precordium and sometimes over back relative to area of coarctation. Adult x-ray examination may show notching of ribs and "3" sign in contour of left upper border of heart.

SAMPLE DOCUMENTATION

Vessels. Neck veins not distended. Both A and V waves are visualized. Jugular venous pressure (JVP) is 4 cm water at 45 degrees. Arterial pulses equal and symmetric, testing on a scale of 1/4.

	C	B	R	F	P	PT	DP
L	2+	2+	2+	2+	2+	2+	2+
R	2+	2+	2+	2+	2+	2+	2+

Vessels soft. No bruits are audible.

Extremities. No edema, skin, or nail changes. Superficial varicosities noted in both lower extremities. No areas of tenderness to palpation.

Blood Pressure Levels for the 90th and 95th Percentiles of Blood Pressure for Boys Aged 1 to 17 Years by Percentiles of Height

Age, Years	Blood Pressure Percentile*	Systolic Blood Pressure by Percentile of Height, mm Hgt							Diastolic Blood Pressure by Percentile of Height, mm Hgt						
		5%	10%	25%	50%	75%	90%	95%	5%	10%	25%	50%	75%	90%	95%
1	90th	94	95	97	98	100	102	102	50	51	52	53	54	54	55
	95th	98	99	101	102	104	106	106	55	55	56	57	58	59	59
2	90th	98	99	100	102	104	105	106	55	55	56	57	58	59	59
	95th	101	102	104	106	108	109	110	59	59	60	61	62	63	63
3	90th	100	101	103	105	107	108	109	59	59	60	61	62	63	63
	95th	104	105	107	109	111	112	113	63	63	64	65	66	67	67
4	90th	102	103	105	107	109	110	111	62	62	63	64	65	66	66
	95th	106	107	109	111	113	114	115	66	67	67	68	69	70	71
5	90th	104	105	106	108	110	112	112	65	65	66	67	68	69	69
	95th	108	109	110	112	114	115	116	69	70	70	71	72	73	74
6	90th	105	106	108	110	111	113	114	67	68	69	70	70	71	72
	95th	109	110	112	114	115	117	117	72	72	73	74	75	76	76
7	90th	106	107	109	111	113	114	115	69	70	71	72	72	73	74
	95th	110	111	113	115	116	118	119	74	74	75	76	77	78	78
8	90th	107	108	110	112	114	115	116	71	71	72	73	74	75	75
	95th	111	112	114	116	118	119	120	75	76	76	77	78	79	80

Age	Percentile														
9	90th	109	110	112	113	115	117	117	72	73	73	74	75	76	77
	95th	113	114	116	117	119	121	121	76	77	78	78	79	80	81
10	90th	110	112	113	115	117	118	119	73	73	74	75	76	77	78
	95th	114	115	117	119	121	122	123	77	78	78	80	80	81	82
11	90th	112	113	115	117	119	120	121	74	74	75	76	77	78	78
	95th	116	117	119	121	123	124	125	78	79	79	80	81	81	83
12	90th	115	116	117	119	121	123	123	75	75	76	76	77	78	79
	95th	119	120	121	123	125	126	127	79	79	80	81	82	82	83
13	90th	117	118	120	122	124	125	126	75	76	76	77	78	79	80
	95th	121	122	124	126	128	129	130	79	79	80	81	82	83	84
14	90th	120	121	123	125	126	128	128	76	76	77	78	79	80	80
	95th	124	125	127	128	130	132	132	80	80	81	82	83	84	85
15	90th	123	124	125	127	129	131	131	77	77	78	79	80	81	81
	95th	127	128	129	131	133	134	135	81	81	82	83	84	85	86
16	90th	125	126	128	130	132	133	134	79	79	80	81	82	82	83
	95th	129	130	132	134	136	137	138	83	83	83	84	85	86	87
17	90th	128	129	131	133	134	136	136	81	81	81	82	83	84	85
	95th	132	133	135	136	138	140	140	85	85	86	87	87	88	89

From Update on task force report on high blood pressure in children, 1996.
*Blood pressure percentile was determined by a single measurement.
†Height percentile was determined by standard growth curves.

Blood Pressure Levels for the 90th and 95th Percentiles of Blood Pressure for Girls Aged 1 to 17 Years by Percentiles of Height

Age, Years	Blood Pressure Percentile*	Systolic Blood Pressure by Percentile of Height, mm Hgt							Diastolic Blood Pressure by Percentile of Height, mm Hgt						
		5%	10%	25%	50%	75%	90%	95%	5%	10%	25%	50%	75%	90%	95%
1	90th	97	98	99	100	102	103	104	53	53	53	54	55	56	56
	95th	101	102	103	104	105	107	107	57	57	57	58	59	60	60
2	90th	99	99	100	102	103	104	105	57	57	58	58	59	60	61
	95th	102	103	104	105	107	108	109	61	61	62	62	63	64	65
3	90th	100	100	102	103	104	105	106	61	61	61	62	63	63	64
	95th	104	104	105	107	108	109	110	65	65	65	66	67	67	68
4	90th	101	102	103	104	106	107	108	63	63	64	65	65	66	67
	95th	105	106	107	108	109	111	111	67	67	68	69	69	70	71
5	90th	103	103	104	106	107	108	109	65	66	66	67	68	68	69
	95th	107	107	108	110	111	112	113	69	70	70	71	72	72	73
6	90th	104	105	106	107	109	110	111	67	67	68	69	69	70	71
	95th	108	109	110	111	112	114	114	71	71	72	73	73	74	75
7	90th	106	107	108	109	110	112	112	69	69	69	70	71	72	72
	95th	110	110	112	113	114	115	116	73	73	73	74	75	76	76
8	90th	108	109	110	111	112	113	114	70	70	71	71	72	73	74
	95th	112	112	113	115	116	117	118	74	74	75	75	76	77	78

Age	BP %ile													
9	90th	110	110	112	113	114	115	116	71	72	73	74	74	75
	95th	114	114	115	117	118	119	120	75	76	77	78	78	79
10	90th	112	112	114	115	116	117	118	73	73	74	75	76	76
	95th	116	116	117	119	120	121	122	77	77	78	79	80	80
11	90th	114	114	116	117	118	119	120	74	75	75	76	77	77
	95th	118	118	119	121	122	123	124	78	79	79	80	81	81
12	90th	116	116	118	119	120	121	122	75	76	76	77	78	78
	95th	120	120	121	123	124	125	126	79	80	80	81	82	82
13	90th	118	118	119	121	122	123	124	76	77	78	78	79	80
	95th	121	122	123	125	126	127	128	80	81	82	82	83	84
14	90th	119	120	121	122	124	125	126	77	78	79	79	80	81
	95th	123	124	125	126	128	129	130	81	82	83	83	84	85
15	90th	121	121	122	124	125	126	127	78	79	80	80	81	82
	95th	124	125	126	128	129	130	131	82	83	84	84	85	86
16	90th	122	122	123	125	126	127	128	79	79	80	81	82	82
	95th	125	126	127	128	130	131	132	83	83	84	85	86	86
17	90th	122	123	124	125	126	128	128	79	79	80	81	82	82
	95th	126	126	127	129	130	131	132	83	83	84	85	86	86

From Update on task force report on high blood pressure in children, 1996.
*Blood pressure percentile was determined by a single measurement.
†Height percentile was determined by standard growth curves.

Clinical and Reference Notes

12

Breasts and Axillae

EQUIPMENT

- Ruler (if mass detected)
- Flashlight with transilluminator (if mass detected)
- Glass slide and cytologic fixative (for nipple discharge)
- Small pillow or folded towel

EXAMINATION

TECHNIQUE	FINDINGS

Females

With patient seated and arms hanging loosely, inspect both breasts

Inspect all quadrants and tail of Spence as shown in figure. If necessary, lift breasts with fingertips to expose lower and lateral aspects.

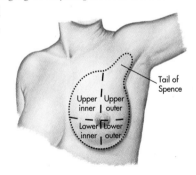

- *Size/shape/symmetry*

EXPECTED: Convex, pendulous, or conical. Frequently asymmetric in size.

TECHNIQUE	FINDINGS
■ *Texture/contour*	**EXPECTED:** Smooth and uninterrupted. **UNEXPECTED:** Dimpling or peau d'orange appearance. Changes or asymmetric appearance.
■ *Skin color*	**EXPECTED:** Consistent color. **UNEXPECTED:** Areas of discoloration or asymmetric appearance.
■ *Venous patterns*	**EXPECTED:** Bilateral venous networks, although pronounced generally only in pregnant or obese women. **UNEXPECTED:** Unilateral network.
■ *Markings*	**EXPECTED:** Long-standing nevi. Supernumerary nipples possible (but could be a clue to other congenital abnormalities). **UNEXPECTED:** Changing or tender nevi. Lesions.
Inspect areolae and nipples	
■ *Size/shape/symmetry*	**EXPECTED:** Areolae round or oval, bilaterally equal or nearly equal. Nipples bilaterally equal or nearly equal in size and usually everted, although one or both sometimes inverted. **UNEXPECTED:** Recent unilateral nipple inversion or retraction.
■ *Color*	**EXPECTED:** Areolae and nipples pink to brown. **UNEXPECTED:** Nonhomogeneous in color.

TECHNIQUE	FINDINGS
■ *Texture/contour*	**EXPECTED:** Areolae smooth, except for Montgomery tubercles. Nipples smooth or wrinkled. **UNEXPECTED:** Areolae with suppurative or tender Montgomery tubercles or with peau d'orange appearance. Nipples crusting, cracking, or with discharge.

With patient in the following positions, reinspect both breasts

■ *Arms extended over head*	**EXPECTED, ALL POSITIONS:** Breasts bilaterally equal with even contour.
■ *Hands pressed on hips or pushed together in front of chest*	**UNEXPECTED:** Dimpling, retraction, deviation, or fixation of breasts.
■ *Seated and leaning over*	
■ *Recumbent*	

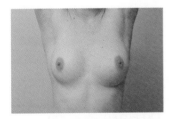
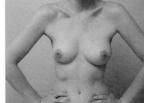
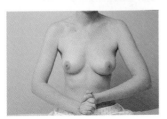
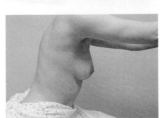

TECHNIQUE   FINDINGS

With patient seated and arms hanging loosely, palpate breasts

First palpate entire breast lightly, then repeat with deeper, heavier palpation. Using finger pads, systematically palpate each breast in all four quadrants and over areolae. Push gently but firmly toward chest while rotating fingers clockwise or counterclockwise, following a *vertical strip, concentric circle,* or *wedge* pattern.

For large breasts, perform bimanual palpation, immobilizing inferior surface with one hand while examining superior surface with the other hand.

EXPECTED: Tissue generally dense, firm, elastic but sometimes lobular. Inframammary ridge may be felt along lower edge of breast. During menstrual cycle, cyclic pattern of breast enlargement, increased nodularity, tenderness.

UNEXPECTED: Lumps or nodules. Characterize any masses by location, size, shape, consistency, tenderness, mobility, delineation of borders, retraction. Use transillumination to assess presence of fluid in masses.

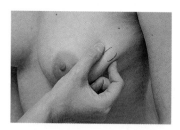

With patient seated and arms raised over her head, palpate tail of Spence

Gently compress tissue between thumb and fingers.

EXPECTED: Similar to expected findings of seated patient, with patient's arms hanging loosely.

UNEXPECTED: Similar to unexpected findings of seated patient, with patient's arms hanging loosely.

TECHNIQUE   FINDINGS

With patient seated and arms flexed at elbows, palpate
for lymph nodes

Right axilla: Support patient's
lower right arm with your
right hand while examining
right axilla with your left
hand. With palmar surface of
fingers, reach deep into hollow, pushing firmly upward;
then bring fingers down, gently rolling soft tissue against
chest wall and axilla. Explore
apex, medial, lateral aspects
along rib cage; lateral aspects
along upper surface of arm;
and anterior and posterior
walls of axilla. Hook fingers
over clavicle and rotate over
supraclavicular area while patient turns head toward same
side and raises shoulder.
Repeat with other axilla.

UNEXPECTED: Nodes, especially in supraclavicular area.
Describe nodes by location,
size, shape, consistency, tenderness, fixation, delineation of
borders.

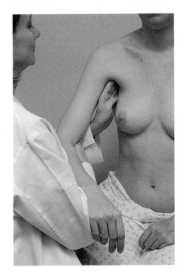

Palpate and compress nipples

Gently compress between
thumb and index finger as
shown.

EXPECTED: Possible nipple
erection and areola puckering.
UNEXPECTED: Discharge.
Note color and origin of any
discharge, and prepare smear.

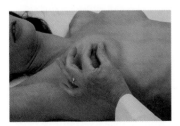

TECHNIQUE	FINDINGS

With patient supine, continue palpation of breast tissue

Have patient put one hand behind head. Place a towel under shoulder of same side. Compress breast tissue between fingers and chest wall, using rotary motion of fingers. Have patient place arm at her side, and repeat palpation. Repeat with other breast.

EXPECTED: Similar to expected findings of patient seated, with arms hanging loosely.

UNEXPECTED: Similar to unexpected findings of patient seated, with arms hanging loosely.

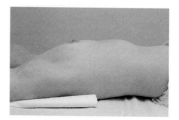

Males

Inspect both breasts

- *Size/shape/symmetry*
- *Surface characteristics*

EXPECTED: Even with chest wall. Sometimes convex (especially in overweight men).
UNEXPECTED: Enlarged breasts.

Inspect areolae and nipples

- *Size/shape/symmetry*

EXPECTED: Areolae round or oval, bilaterally equal or nearly equal. Nipples bilaterally equal or nearly equal in size and usually everted, although one or both sometimes inverted.
UNEXPECTED: Recent unilateral nipple inversion or retraction.

- *Color*

EXPECTED: Areolae and nipples pink to brown.
UNEXPECTED: Nonhomogeneous in color.

TECHNIQUE	FINDINGS
■ *Texture/contour*	**EXPECTED:** Areolae smooth, except for Montgomery tubercles. Nipples smooth or wrinkled. **UNEXPECTED:** Areolae with suppurative or tender Montgomery tubercles or with peau d'orange appearance. Nipples crusting, cracking, or with discharge.

Palpate breasts and over areolae

| Palpate briefly, following palpation steps for females. | **EXPECTED:** Thin layer of fatty tissue overlying muscle. Thick layer in obese men may give appearance of breast enlargement. Firm disk of glandular tissue sometimes evident.
UNEXPECTED: Lumps or nodules. |

With patient seated and arms flexed at elbows, palpate for lymph nodes

| Palpate as described for females. | **UNEXPECTED:** Nodes, especially in supraclavicular area. Describe nodes by location, size, shape, consistency, tenderness, fixation, delineation of borders. |

Palpate and compress nipples

| Gently compress between thumb and index finger. | **EXPECTED:** Possible nipple erection and areola puckering.
UNEXPECTED: Discharge. Note color and origin of any discharge, and prepare smear. |

AIDS TO DIFFERENTIAL DIAGNOSIS

ABNORMALITY	DESCRIPTION
Fibrocystic disease Fibroadenoma Malignant breast tumors	See table of differentiating signs and symptoms, p. 139.
Adult gynecomastia	Smooth, firm, mobile, tender disk of breast tissue behind areola in males, unilaterally or bilaterally.
Mastitis	Swelling, tenderness, heat; patient may have fever. Abscess—pus-filled, hardened mass that is fluctuant, hard, erythematous.

PEDIATRIC VARIATIONS

EXAMINATION

TECHNIQUE	FINDINGS
Palpate and compress nipples	
	EXPECTED: Breast enlargement is not unusual in newborns. "Witch's milk" may be expressed.

AIDS TO DIFFERENTIAL DIAGNOSIS

ABNORMALITY	DESCRIPTION
Gynecomastia	Enlargement of breast tissue in boys caused by puberty, hormonal imbalance, testicular or pituitary tumors, or medications containing estrogens or steroids. Thorough investigation should be conducted to rule out pathologic conditions.

Differentiating Signs and Symptoms of Breast Masses

	Fibrocystic Disease	Fibroadenoma	Cancer
Age, years	20-49	15-55	30-80
Occurrence	Usually bilateral	Usually bilateral	Usually unilateral
Number	Multiple or single	Single; may be multiple	Single
Shape	Round	Round or discoid	Irregular or stellate
Consistency	Soft to firm; tense	Firm, rubbery	Hard, stonelike
Mobility	Mobile	Mobile	Fixed
Retraction signs	Absent	Absent	Often present
Tenderness	Usually tender	Usually nontender	Usually nontender
Delimitation	Well delineated	Well delineated	Poorly delineated; irregular
Variation with menses	Yes	No	No

SAMPLE DOCUMENTATION

Females

Subjective. A 42-year-old female who noticed a "knot" in her right lower breast last week. Denies nipple discharge or skin changes. Reports normal mammogram 2 years ago. Has never had a breast lump before. Currently on last day of menses. Has breast tenderness just before menses but denies breast pain today. No family history of breast cancer.

Objective. Breasts moderate size, conical shape, left slightly larger than right. No skin lesions, contour smooth without dimpling or retraction; venous pattern symmetric. Nipple symmetric, without discharge; Montgomery tubercles bilaterally. Tissue dense, particularly in upper quadrants; 3×2 cm soft mass in lower left quadrant of right breast. Mobile, nontender. No nipple discharge expressed. No supraclavicular, infraclavicular, or axillary lymphadenopathy.

13

Abdomen

EQUIPMENT

- Stethoscope
- Skin-marking pencil
- Centimeter ruler or tape measure
- Reflex hammer or tongue blade

EXAMINATION

Have patient in the supine position to start the examination.

TECHNIQUE	FINDINGS
Inspect abdomen in all four quadrants (see box on p. 142)	
■ *Skin color/characteristics*	**EXPECTED:** Usual color variations, such as paleness or tanning lines. Fine venous network (venous return toward head above umbilicus, toward feet below umbilicus).
	UNEXPECTED: Generalized color changes, such as jaundice or cyanosis. Glistening taut appearance. Bluish periumbilical discoloration, bruises, other localized discoloration. Striae, lesions or nodules, a pearl-like enlarged umbilical node, scars.

141

Anatomic Correlates of the Four Quadrants of the Abdomen

Right Upper Quadrant	Left Upper Quadrant
Liver and gallbladder	Left lobe of liver
Pylorus	Spleen
Duodenum	Stomach
Head of pancreas	Body of pancreas
Right adrenal gland	Left adrenal gland
Portion of right kidney	Portion of left kidney
Hepatic flexure of colon	Splenic flexure of colon
Portions of ascending and transverse colon	Portions of transverse and descending colon
Right Lower Quadrant	**Left Lower Quadrant**
Lower pole of right kidney	Lower pole of left kidney
Cecum and appendix	Sigmoid colon
Portion of ascending colon	Portion of descending colon
Bladder (if distended)	Bladder (if distended)
Ovary and salpinx	Ovary and salpinx
Uterus (if enlarged)	Uterus (if enlarged)
Right spermatic cord	Left spermatic cord
Right ureter	Left ureter

From Barkauskas, 2001.

TECHNIQUE

FINDINGS

- *Contour/symmetry*

  Begin seated to patient's right to enhance shadows and contouring. Inspect while patient breathes comfortably and while patient holds a deep breath. Assess symmetry, first seated at patient's side, then standing behind patient's head.

EXPECTED: Flat, rounded, or scaphoid. Contralateral areas symmetric. Maximum height of convexity at umbilicus. Abdomen remains smooth and symmetric while patient holds breath.

UNEXPECTED: Umbilicus displaced upward, downward, or laterally or is inflamed, swollen, or bulging. Any distention (symmetric or asymmetric), bulges, or masses while breathing comfortably or holding breath.

TECHNIQUE	FINDINGS
■ *Surface motion*	**EXPECTED:** Smooth, even motion with respiration. Females mostly costal; males mostly abdominal. Pulsation in upper midline in thin adults. **UNEXPECTED:** Limited motion with respiration in adult males. Rippling movement (peristalsis) or marked pulsation.

Inspect abdominal muscles as patient raises head

EXPECTED: No masses or protrusions.
UNEXPECTED: Masses, protrusion of the umbilicus and other hernia signs, or muscle separation.

Auscultate with stethoscope diaphragm

■ *Frequency and character of bowel sounds*
Warm stethoscope diaphragm, and hold with light pressure. Auscultate in all quadrants.

EXPECTED: 5 to 35 irregular clicks and gurgles per minute. Borborygmi or increased sounds due to hunger.
UNEXPECTED: Increased sounds unrelated to hunger, high-pitched tinkling, or decreased or absent sounds after 5 minutes of listening.

■ *Liver and spleen*

EXPECTED: Silent.
UNEXPECTED: Friction rubs.

Auscultate with stethoscope bell

■ *Vascular sounds*
Listen with stethoscope bell in all quadrants.

EXPECTED: No bruits, venous hum, or friction rubs.
UNEXPECTED: Bruits in aortic, renal, iliac, or femoral arteries.

TECHNIQUE	FINDINGS

- *Epigastric region and around umbilicus*

EXPECTED: No venous hum.
UNEXPECTED: Venous hum.

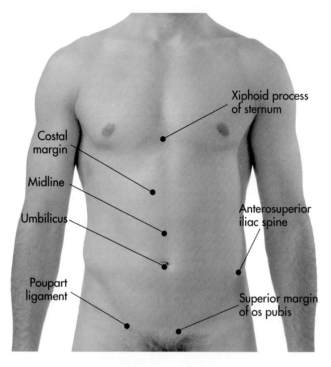

From Thompson and Wilson, 1996.

Percussion Notes of the Abdomen

Note	Description	Location
Tympany	Musical note of higher pitch than resonance	Over air-filled viscera
Hyperresonance	Pitch lies between tympany and resonance	Base of left lung
Resonance	Sustained note of moderate pitch	Over lung tissue and sometimes over abdomen
Dullness	Short, high-pitched note with little resonance	Over solid organs adjacent to air-filled structures

Modified from AH Robins Co.

TECHNIQUE	FINDINGS

Percuss abdomen

NOTE: Percussion can be done independently or concurrently with palpation.

- *Tone*
Percuss in all quadrants.

EXPECTED: Tympany predominant. Dullness over organs and solid masses. Dullness in suprapubic area from distended bladder. See table on p. 144 for percussion notes.

UNEXPECTED: Dullness predominant.

- *Liver span*
To determine lower liver border, percuss upward at right midclavicular line, as shown in figure, and mark with a pen where tympany changes to dullness. To determine upper liver border, percuss downward at right midclavicular line from an area of resonance, and mark change to dullness. Measure the distance between marks to estimate vertical span.

EXPECTED: Lower border usually begins at or slightly below costal margin. Upper border usually begins at fifth to seventh intercostal space. Span generally ranges from 6 to 12 cm in adults.

UNEXPECTED: Lower liver border more than 2 to 3 cm below costal margin. Upper liver border below seventh or above fifth intercostal span. Span greater than 12 cm or less than 6 cm.

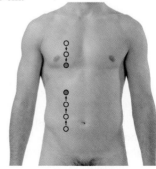

From Thompson and Wilson, 1996.

TECHNIQUE	FINDINGS

■ *Spleen*

Percuss just posterior to midaxillary line on left, beginning at areas of lung resonance and moving in several directions. Percuss lowest intercostal space in left anterior axillary line before and after patient takes deep breath.

EXPECTED: Small area of dullness from sixth to tenth rib. Tympany before and after deep breath.
UNEXPECTED: Large area of dullness (check for full stomach or feces-filled intestine). Tone change from tympany to dullness with inspiration.

■ *Stomach*

Percuss in area of left lower anterior rib cage and left epigastric region.

EXPECTED: Tympany of gastric air bubble (lower than intestine tympany).
UNEXPECTED: Dullness.

Lightly palpate abdomen

Stand at patient's side (usually right). Systematically palpate all quadrants, avoiding areas previously identified as trouble spots. With palmar surfaces of fingers, depress abdominal wall up to 1 cm with light, even motion. Identify areas of peritoneal irritation by assessing for cutaneous hypersensitivity.

EXPECTED: Abdomen smooth with consistent softness. Possible tension from palpating too deeply, cold hands, or ticklishness.
UNEXPECTED: Muscular tension or resistance, tenderness, or masses. If resistance is present, place pillow under patient's knees, and ask patient to breathe slowly through mouth. Feel for relaxation of rectus abdominis muscles on expiration. Continuing tension signals involuntary response to abdominal rigidity. Cutaneous hypersensitivity.

Palpate abdomen with moderate pressure

Using same hand position as above, palpate all quadrants again, this time with moderate pressure.

EXPECTED: Soft, nontender.
UNEXPECTED: Tenderness.

TECHNIQUE   FINDINGS

Deeply palpate abdomen

With same hand position as above, repeat palpation in all quadrants, pressing deeply and evenly into abdominal wall. Move fingers back and forth over abdominal contents. Use bimanual technique—exerting pressure with top hand and concentrating on sensation with bottom hand, as shown in figure at right—if obesity or muscular resistance makes deep palpation difficult. To help determine whether masses are superficial or intraabdominal, have patient lift head from examining table to contract abdominal muscles and obscure intraabdominal masses.

EXPECTED: Possible sensation of abdominal wall sliding back and forth. Possible awareness of borders of rectus abdominis muscles, aorta, and portions of colon. Possible tenderness over cecum, sigmoid colon, and aorta and in midline near xiphoid process.

UNEXPECTED: Bulges, masses, tenderness unrelated to deep palpation of cecum, sigmoid colon, aorta, xiphoid process. Note location, size, shape, consistency, tenderness, pulsation, mobility, movement (with respiration) of any masses.

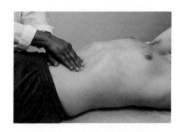

From Thompson and Wilson, 1996.

■ *Umbilical ring and umbilicus*
Palpate umbilical ring and around umbilicus. Note whether ring is incomplete or soft in center.

EXPECTED: Umbilical ring circular and free of irregularities. Umbilicus either slightly inverted or everted.

UNEXPECTED: Bulges, nodules, granulation. Protruding umbilicus.

TECHNIQUE	FINDINGS

- *Liver*
  Place left hand under patient at eleventh and twelfth ribs, lifting to elevate liver toward abdominal wall. Place right hand on abdomen, fingers extended toward head with tips on right midclavicular line below level of liver dullness, as shown in figure at right. Alternatively, place right hand parallel to right costal margin, as shown in figure at right, below. Press right hand gently but deeply in and up. Ask patient to breathe comfortably a few times and then take a deep breath. Feel for liver edge as diaphragm pushes it down. If palpable, repeat maneuver medially and laterally to costal margin.

  EXPECTED: Usually liver is not palpable. If felt, liver edge should be firm, smooth, even.
  UNEXPECTED: Tenderness, nodules, or irregularity.

  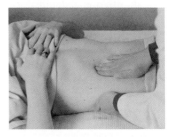

  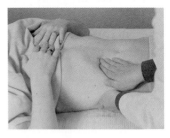

  From Thompson and Wilson, 1996.

- *Gallbladder*
  Palpate below liver margin at lateral border of rectus abdominis muscle.

  EXPECTED: Gallbladder not palpable.
  UNEXPECTED: Palpable, tender or nontender. If tender (possible cholecystitis), palpate deeply during inspiration and observe for pain (Murphy sign).

TECHNIQUE   FINDINGS

■ *Spleen*
Reach across patient with left
hand, place it beneath patient
over left costovertebral angle,
and lift spleen anteriorly toward abdominal wall. As
shown in figure, place right
hand on abdomen below left
costal margin and—using
findings from percussion—
gently press fingertips inward
toward spleen while asking
patient to take a deep breath.
Feel for spleen as it moves
downward toward fingers.
Repeat with patient lying on
right side, as shown in figure
below, with hips and knees
flexed. Press inward with left
hand while using fingertips
of right hand to feel edge of
spleen.

EXPECTED: Spleen usually not
palpable by either method.
UNEXPECTED: Palpable
spleen.

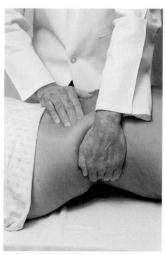

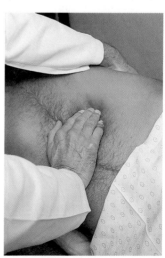

TECHNIQUE	FINDINGS

- *Left kidney*
  Standing on patient's right, reach across with left hand, and place over left flank; then place right hand at patient's left costal margin. Ask patient to inhale deeply, while you elevate left flank and palpate deeply with right hand.

EXPECTED: Left kidney usually not palpable.
UNEXPECTED: Pain.

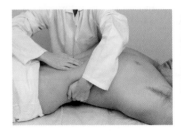

- *Right kidney*
  Standing on patient's right, place left hand under right flank, then place right hand at patient's right costal margin. Ask patient to inhale deeply while you elevate right flank and palpate deeply with right hand.

EXPECTED: If palpable, right kidney should be smooth and firm with rounded edges.
UNEXPECTED: Tenderness.

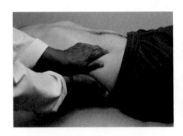

From Thompson and Wilson, 1996.

- *Aorta*
  Palpate deeply slightly to left of midline, and feel for aortic pulsation. As an alternative technique, place palmar surface of hands with fingers extended on midline; press fingers deeply inward on each side of aorta, and feel for pulsation. For thin patients, use one hand, placing thumb and fingers on either side of aorta.

EXPECTED: Pulsation anterior in direction.
UNEXPECTED: Prominent lateral pulsation.

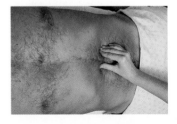

TECHNIQUE	FINDINGS

■ *Urinary bladder*
Percuss distended bladder to help determine outline, then palpate.

EXPECTED: Ordinarily not palpable unless distended with urine. If distended, bladder should be smooth, round, and tense and on percussion will elicit lower note than surrounding air-filled intestines.
UNEXPECTED: Palpable when not distended with urine.

Elicit abdominal reflexes

Stroke each quadrant of abdomen with end of reflex hammer or tongue blade edge. Elicit upper abdominal reflexes by stroking upward and away from umbilicus; elicit lower abdominal reflexes by stroking downward and away from umbilicus.

EXPECTED: With each stroke, contraction of rectus abdominis muscles and pulling of umbilicus toward stroked side. Reflex may be diminished in patient who is obese or whose abdominal muscles were stretched during pregnancy.
UNEXPECTED: Absence of reflex.

With patient sitting, percuss costovertebral angles

Stand behind patient. *Right side:* Place left hand over right costovertebral angle and strike with ulnar surface of left fist. *Left side:* Repeat with hands reversed.

EXPECTED: No tenderness.
UNEXPECTED: Kidney tenderness or pain.

Pain assessment

Keep eyes on patient's face while examining abdomen. To help characterize pain, have patient cough, take a deep breath, jump, or walk. Ask whether patient is hungry.

UNEXPECTED: Unwillingness to move, nausea, vomiting, areas of localized tenderness. Lack of hunger. See box and table on p. 152.

Some Causes of Pain Perceived in Anatomic Regions

Right Upper Quadrant
Duodenal ulcer
Hepatitis
Hepatomegaly
Pneumonia

Right Lower Quadrant
Appendicitis
Salpingitis
Ovarian cyst
Ruptured ectopic pregnancy
Renal/ureteral stone
Strangulated hernia
Meckel diverticulitis
Regional ileitis
Perforated cecum

Periumbilical
Intestinal obstruction
Acute pancreatitis
Early appendicitis
Mesenteric thrombosis
Aortic aneurysm
Diverticulitis

Left Upper Quadrant
Ruptured spleen
Gastric ulcer
Aortic aneurysm
Perforated colon
Pneumonia

Left Lower Quadrant
Sigmoid diverticulitis
Salpingitis
Ovarian cyst
Ruptured ectopic pregnancy
Renal/ureteral stone
Strangulated hernia
Perforated colon
Regional ileitis
Ulcerative colitis

Modified from Judge et al, 1988.

Quality and Onset of Abdominal Pain

Characteristic	Possible Related Condition
Burning	Peptic ulcer
Cramping	Biliary colic, gastroenteritis
Colic	Appendicitis with impacted feces; renal stone
Aching	Appendiceal irritation
Knifelike	Pancreatitis
Gradual onset	Infection
Sudden onset	Duodenal ulcer, acute pancreatitis, obstruction, perforation

TECHNIQUE	FINDINGS

Iliopsoas muscle test

Use test for suspected appendicitis. With patient supine, place hand over lower thigh. Ask patient to raise leg, flexing at hip, while you push downward.

UNEXPECTED: Lower quadrant pain.

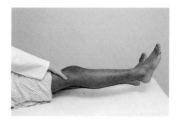

Obturator muscle test

Use test for suspected ruptured appendix or pelvic abscess. With patient supine, ask patient to flex right leg at hip and bend knee to 90 degrees. Hold leg just above knee, grasp ankle, and rotate leg laterally and medially, as shown in figure at right.

UNEXPECTED: Pain in hypogastric region.

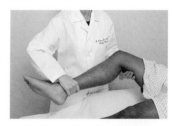

AIDS TO DIFFERENTIAL DIAGNOSIS

ABNORMALITY	DESCRIPTION
Hiatal hernia with esophagitis	Epigastric pain and/or heartburn that worsens with reclining and is relieved by sitting or with antacids; water brash; or dysphagia. Sudden onset of vomiting, pain, complete dysphagia are symptoms of hernia incarceration.

ABNORMALITY	DESCRIPTION
Gastroesophageal reflux disease (GERD)	Backward flow of acid from stomach up into esophagus. Patients may experience heartburn, a sour taste of acid in the back of the throat, or hoarseness. Symptoms in infants and children include regurgitation and vomiting. Condition can cause respiratory problems from aspiration and bleeding from esophagitis.
Duodenal ulcer	Localized epigastric pain occurring with empty stomach that is relieved with food or antacids. Tenderness on palpation of abdomen for anterior-wall ulcers. Hematemesis, melena, dizziness or syncope, decreased blood pressure, increased pulse rate, decreased hematocrit level are symptoms of upper gastrointestinal (GI) bleeding. Signs of an acute abdomen could indicate perforation of duodenum, **a life-threatening event.**
Crohn disease	Cramping diarrhea, mild bleeding, occurs anywhere in GI tract; fissure, fistula abscess formation; periumbilical colic; malabsorption; folate deficiency.
Ulcerative colitis	Mild to severe symptoms; bloody, watery diarrhea; no localized peritoneal signs; weight loss, fatigue, general debility.

Abdominal Signs Associated With Common Abnormalities

Sign	Description	Associated Conditions
Aaron	Pain or distress occurs in the area of patient's heart or stomach on palpation of McBurney point	Appendicitis
Ballance	Fixed dullness to percussion in left flank and dullness in right flank that disappears on change of position	Peritoneal irritation
Blumberg	Rebound tenderness	Peritoneal irritation, appendicitis
Cullen	Ecchymosis around umbilicus	Hemoperitoneum, pancreatitis, ectopic pregnancy
Dance	Absence of bowel sounds in right lower quadrant	Intussusception
Grey Turner	Ecchymosis of flanks	Hemoperitoneum, pancreatitis
Kehr	Abdominal pain radiating to left shoulder	Spleen rupture, renal calculi, ectopic pregnancy
Markle (heel jar)	Patient stands with straightened knees, then raises up on toes, relaxes, and allows heels to hit floor, thus jarring body; action will cause abdominal pain if positive	Peritoneal irritation, appendicitis
McBurney	Rebound tenderness and sharp pain when McBurney point is palpated	Appendicitis
Murphy	Abrupt cessation of inspiration on palpation of gallbladder	Cholecystitis
Romberg-Howship	Pain down medial aspect of thigh to knees	Strangulated obturator hernia
Rovsing	Right lower quadrant pain intensified by left lower quadrant abdominal palpation	Peritoneal irritation, appendicitis

ABNORMALITY	DESCRIPTION
Irritable bowel syndrome (IBS)	Functional disorder of the intestine that produces a cluster of symptoms, usually abdominal pain, bloating, constipation, diarrhea. Some patients with IBS experience alternating diarrhea and constipation. Mucus may be present around or within the stool.
Colon cancer	Occult blood in stool. History of changes in frequency or character of stool. Lesion felt on rectal examination. Tumor palpated in right or left lower quadrant.
Hepatitis	Jaundice, anorexia, abdominal gastric discomfort, clay-colored stools, tea-colored urine. Enlarged liver. Caused by viral infection, alcohol, drugs, or toxins.
Cirrhosis	Ascites, jaundice, prominent abdominal vasculature, cutaneous spider angiomas, dark urine, light-colored stools, spleen enlargement. Complaints of fatigue. Muscle wasting in late stages.
Cholecystitis	*Acute:* Pain in upper right quadrant with radiation around midtorso to right scapular region. Pain abrupt and severe, lasting 2 to 4 hours. *Chronic:* Repeated acute attacks; a scarred and contracted gallbladder; fat intolerance, flatulence, nausea, anorexia, nonspecific abdominal pain and tenderness of right hypochondriac region.

ABNORMALITY	DESCRIPTION
Chronic pancreatitis	Unremitting abdominal pain, epigastric tenderness, weight loss, steatorrhea, glucose intolerance.
Pyelonephritis	Flank pain, bacteriuria, pyuria, dysuria, nocturia, urinary frequency. Possible costovertebral angle tenderness.
Renal calculi	Fever, hematuria, flank pain that may extend to groin and genitals.
Appendicitis	Initially, periumbilical or epigastric pain; colicky; later becomes localized to right lower quadrant, often at McBurney point.

PEDIATRIC VARIATIONS

EXAMINATION

TECHNIQUE	FINDINGS
Inspect abdomen in all four quadrants	
Infant's abdomen should be examined, if possible, during a time of relaxation and quiet. Sucking on a bottle or pacifier may help to relax infant.	
■ Contour/symmetry	**EXPECTED:** Until the age of 3 years, children's abdomens will protrude when standing.
■ Surface motion	**EXPECTED:** Pulsation in epigastric area in infants. **UNEXPECTED:** Peristaltic waves associated with pyloric stenosis.
Percuss abdomen	
■ Tone	**EXPECTED:** More tympany is present in children than adults.

Differential Diagnosis of Urinary Incontinence

Condition	History	Physical Findings
Stress incontinence	Small-volume incontinence with coughing, sneezing, laughing, running; history of prior pelvic surgery	Pelvic floor relaxation; cystocele, rectocele; lax urethral sphincter; loss of urine with provocative testing; atrophic vaginitis; postvoid residual <100 ml
Urge incontinence	Uncontrolled urge to void; large-volume incontinence; history of central nervous system (CNS) disorders such as stroke, multiple sclerosis, parkinsonism	Unexpected findings only as related to CNS disorder; postvoid residual <100 ml
Overflow incontinence	Small-volume incontinence, dribbling, hesitancy; in men symptoms of enlarged prostate—nocturia, dribbling, hesitancy, deceased force and caliber of stream	Distended bladder; prostate hypertrophy; stool in rectum, fecal impaction; postvoid residual >100 ml
bance	In neurogenic bladder—history of bowel problems, spinal cord injury, or multiple sclerosis	Evidence of spinal cord disease or diabetic neuropathy; lax sphincter; gait distur-
Functional incontinence	Change in mental status, impaired mobility, new environment	Impaired mental status; impaired mobility
	Medications—hypnotics, diuretics, anti-cholinergic agents, α-adrenergic agents, calcium channel blockers	Impaired mental status or unexpected find-ings only as related to other physical con-ditions

TECHNIQUE	FINDINGS
Deeply palpate abdomen	
■ *Umbilical ring*	**EXPECTED:** Children up to 4 years old may have an umbilical hernia.
■ *Liver*	**EXPECTED:** Liver may be palpable in young children 2 to 3 cm below costal margin.

AGE	LIVER SPAN (CM)
6 months	2.4-2.8
12 months	2.8-3.1
24 months	3.5-3.6
3 years	4.0
4 years	4.3-4.4
5 years	4.5-5.1
6 years	4.8-5.1
8 years	5.1-5.6
10 years	5.5-6.1

SAMPLE DOCUMENTATION

Subjective. A 44-year-old female complains of burning sensation in epigastric area and chest. Occurs after eating, especially with spicy foods. Lasts 1 to 2 hours and is worse when lying down. Sometimes causes bitter taste in mouth. Also feels bloated. Antacids do not relieve symptoms. Denies nausea/vomiting/diarrhea. No cough or shortness of breath.

Abdomen. Abdomen rounded and symmetric, with white striae adjacent to umbilicus in all quadrants. A well-healed 5-cm white surgical scar evident in right lower quadrant. No areas of visible pulsations or peristalsis. Active bowel sounds audible in all four quadrants. Percussion tones tympanic over epigastrium and resonant over remainder of abdomen. Liver span 8 cm at right midclavicular line. On inspiration, liver edge firm, smooth, nontender. No splenomegaly. Musculature soft and relaxed to light palpation. No masses or areas of tenderness to deep palpation. Superficial reflexes intact. No costovertebral angle tenderness.

Clinical and Reference Notes

14

Female Genitalia

EQUIPMENT

- Gloves
- Sterile cotton swabs
- Culture plates
- Cytologic fixative
- Speculum
- Water-soluble lubricant

- Lamp
- Wooden or plastic spatula
- Glass slides
- Cervical brushes
- DNA probe kits for *Chlamydia*/gonorrhea

EXAMINATION

Have patient in lithotomy position, draped for minimal exposure.

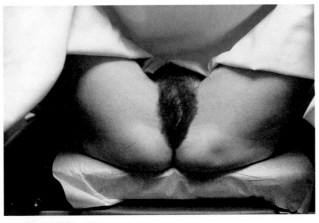

From Edge and Miller, 1994.

TECHNIQUE   FINDINGS

External Genitalia

Wear gloves on both hands

Ask patient to separate or drop open her knees. Tell patient you are beginning examination, then touch either lower thigh and—without breaking contact—move hand along thigh to external genitalia.

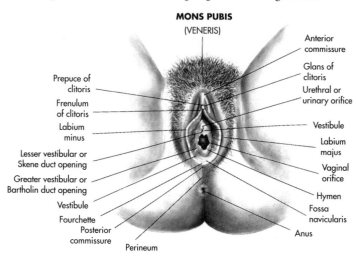

From Lowdermilk et al, 1997.

Inspect and palpate mons pubis

■ *Characteristics*

EXPECTED: Skin smooth and clean.
UNEXPECTED: Improper hygiene.

■ *Pubic hair*

EXPECTED: Regularly distributed female pubic hair.
UNEXPECTED: Nits or lice.

Inspect and palpate labia

■ *Labia majora*

EXPECTED: Gaping or closed, dry or moist, shriveled or full, tissue soft and homogeneous, usually symmetric.

TECHNIQUE	FINDINGS

| | **UNEXPECTED:** Swelling, redness, tenderness, discoloration, varicosities, obvious stretching, or signs of trauma or scarring. If excoriation, rashes, or lesions are present, ask patient whether she has been scratching. |

- *Labia minora*
  Separate labia majora with fingers of one hand. With other hand, palpate labia minora between thumb and second finger.

EXPECTED: Moist, dark-pink inner surface. Tissue soft and homogeneous.

UNEXPECTED: Tenderness, inflammation, irritation, excoriation, caking of discharge in tissue folds, discoloration, ulcers, vesicles, irregularities, or nodules. Hyperemia of fourchette not related to recent sexual activity.

Inspect clitoris
- *Size and length*

EXPECTED: Length 2 cm or less; diameter 0.5 cm.

UNEXPECTED: Enlargement, atrophy, inflammation, or adhesions.

Inspect urethral meatus and vaginal opening
- *Urethral orifice*

EXPECTED: Slit or irregular opening, close to or in vaginal introitus, usually midline.

UNEXPECTED: Discharge, polyps, caruncles, fistulas, lesions, irritation, inflammation, or dilation.

TECHNIQUE	FINDINGS
■ *Vaginal introitus*	**EXPECTED:** Thin vertical slit or large orifice with irregular edges. Tissue moist. **UNEXPECTED:** Swelling, discoloration, discharge, lesions, fistulas, or fissures.

Milk Skene glands

Tell patient you will be inserting one finger in her vagina and pressing forward with it. With palm up, insert index finger to second joint, press upward, and milk Skene glands by moving finger outward. Perform on both sides of urethra and directly on urethra.

UNEXPECTED: Discharge or tenderness. Note color, consistency, odor of any discharge; obtain culture.

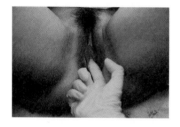

From Edge and Miller, 1994.

Palpate Bartholin glands

Tell patient she will feel you pressing around entrance to vagina. Palpate lateral tissue between index finger and thumb, then palpate entire area bilaterally, particularly posterolateral portion of labia majora.

EXPECTED: No swelling.
UNEXPECTED: Swelling, tenderness, masses, heat, fluctuation, or discharge. Note color, consistency, odor of any discharge; obtain culture.

Test vaginal muscle tone if indicated

Ask patient to squeeze vaginal opening around your finger.

EXPECTED: Fairly tight squeezing by some nulliparous women, less so by some multiparous women.
UNEXPECTED: Protrusion of cervix or uterus.

TECHNIQUE	FINDINGS

Inspect for bulging and urinary incontinence

Ask patient to bear down.

EXPECTED: No bulging.
UNEXPECTED: Bulging of anterior or posterior wall, or urinary incontinence.

Inspect and palpate perineum

Compress perineum tissue between finger and thumb.

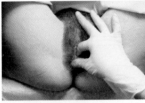

From Edge and Miller, 1994.

EXPECTED: Perineum surface smooth—generally thick and smooth in a nulliparous woman, thinner and rigid in a multiparous woman. Possible episiotomy scarring in women who have borne children.
UNEXPECTED: Tenderness, inflammation, fistulas, lesions, or growths.

Inspect anus

■ *Skin characteristics*

EXPECTED: Skin darkly pigmented and possibly coarse.
UNEXPECTED: Scarring, lesions, inflammation, fissures, lumps, skin tags, or excoriation.

Internal Genitalia—Speculum Examination

If you touched the perineum or anal skin while examining the external genitalia, change gloves before beginning internal examination.

Lubricate speculum and gloved fingers with water (if you expect to take specimens for analysis) or water-soluble lubricant (if you do not).

TECHNIQUE   FINDINGS

Insert speculum

Tell patient she will feel you
touching her again, then insert
two fingers of hand not holding
the speculum just inside vaginal
introitus and press downward.
Ask patient to breathe slowly
and try to consciously relax her
muscles. Use fingers of that
hand to separate labia minora

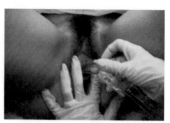

From Edge and Miller, 1994.

widely so that hymenal opening
becomes clearly visible. Then
slowly insert speculum along
path of least resistance, often
slightly downward, avoiding
trauma to urethra and vaginal
walls. Some clinicians insert
speculum blades at an oblique
angle; others prefer to keep
blades horizontal. In either case
avoid touching clitoris, catching
pubic hair, or pinching labial
skin. Insert speculum the

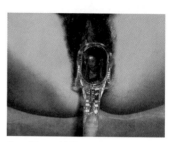

From Edge and Miller, 1994.

length of the vaginal canal.
Maintaining downward pressure, open speculum by pressing on thumb piece. Sweep
speculum slowly upward until
cervix comes into view. Adjust
light, then manipulate speculum farther into vagina so that
cervix is well exposed between
anterior and posterior blades.
Stabilize distal spread of blades,
and adjust proximal spread as
needed.

TECHNIQUE	FINDINGS

Inspect cervix

■ *Color*

EXPECTED: Evenly distributed pink. Symmetric, circumscribed erythema around os can be expected.

UNEXPECTED: Bluish, pale, or reddened cervix (especially if patchy or with irregular borders).

■ *Position*

EXPECTED: In midline, horizontal or pointing anteriorly or posteriorly. Protruding into vagina 1 to 3 cm.

UNEXPECTED: Deviation to right or left. Protrusion into vagina greater than 1 to 3 cm.

■ *Size*

EXPECTED: 3 cm in diameter.

UNEXPECTED: Larger than 3 cm.

■ *Shape*

EXPECTED: Uniform.

UNEXPECTED: Distorted.

■ *Surface characteristics*

EXPECTED: Surface smooth. Possible symmetric, reddened circle around os (squamo-columnar epithelium). Possible small, white, or yellow, raised round areas on cervix (nabothian cysts).

UNEXPECTED: Friable tissue, red patchy areas, granular areas, or white patches.

■ *Discharge*
Note any discharge.
Determine origin—cervix or vagina.

EXPECTED: Odorless, creamy or clear, thick, thin, or stringy (often heavier at midcycle or immediately before menstruation).

UNEXPECTED: Odorous and white to yellow, green, or gray.

TECHNIQUE	FINDINGS

■ *Size and shape of os*
Follow standard precautions for safe collection of human secretions.

EXPECTED: *Nulliparous woman:* Small, round, oval. *Multiparous woman:* Usually a horizontal slit or irregular and stellate.

UNEXPECTED: Slit resulting from trauma from induced abortion, difficult removal of intrauterine device (IUD), or sexual abuse.

Withdraw speculum, and inspect vaginal walls

Unlock speculum, and remove it slowly, rotating it so vaginal walls can be inspected.

Maintain downward pressure, and hook index finger over anterior blade as it is removed. Note odor of any discharge pooled in posterior blade, and obtain specimen if not already obtained.

EXPECTED: Vaginal wall color same pink as cervix or lighter; moist, smooth or rugated; and homogeneous. Thin, clear or cloudy, odorless secretions.

UNEXPECTED: Reddened patches, lesions, pallor, cracks, bleeding, nodules, swelling. Secretions that are profuse; thick, curdy, or frothy; gray, green, or yellow; or malodorous.

Internal Genitalia—Bimanual Examination

Change gloves, and then lubricate index and middle fingers of examining hand.

Tell patient you are going to examine her internally with your fingers. Prevent thumb from touching clitoris during examination.

Palpate vaginal wall while inserting fingers into vagina

Insert tips of index and middle fingers into vaginal opening and press downward, waiting for muscles to relax. Gradually insert fingers full length while palpating vaginal wall.

EXPECTED: Smooth and homogeneous.

UNEXPECTED: Tenderness, lesions, cysts, nodules, masses, or growths.

Obtaining Vaginal Smears and Cultures

Vaginal specimens are obtained while the speculum is in place in the vagina but after the cervix and its surrounding tissue have been inspected. Collect specimens as indicated for a Papanicolaou (Pap) smear, sexually transmitted disease screening, and wet mount. Label the specimen with the patient's name and a description of the specimen (e.g., cervical smear, vaginal smear, and culture). Be sure to follow standard precautions for the safe collection of human secretions.

Pap Smear

Brushes are now being used in conjunction with, or instead of, the conventional spatula to improve the quality of cells obtained. The cylindric-type brush (e.g., a Cytobrush) collects endocervical cells only. First, collect a sample from the ectocervix with a spatula. Insert the longer projection of the spatula into the cervical os. Rotate it 360 degrees, keeping it flush against the cervical tissue. Withdraw the spatula, and spread the specimen on a glass slide. A single light stroke with each side of the spatula is sufficient to thin out the specimen over the slide. Immediately spray with cytologic fixative, and label the slide as the ectocervical specimen. Then introduce the brush device into the vagina, and insert it into the cervical os until only the bristles closest to the handle are exposed. Slowly rotate one half to one full turn. Remove and prepare the endocervical smear by rolling and twisting the brush with moderate pressure across a glass slide. Fix the specimen with spray, and label as the endocervical specimen.

For the ThinPrep technology procedure utilizing the Cytobrush/plastic spatula combination, obtain an adequate sampling from the ectocervix using the plastic spatula. Rinse the spatula into the solution vial by swirling the spatula vigorously in the vial 10 times. Discard the spatula. Obtain an adequate sampling from the endocervix using an endocervical brush device. Insert the brush into the cervix until only the bottommost fibers are exposed. Slowly rotate one-fourth or one-half turn in one direction. Do not overrotate. Rinse the brush into the solution vial by rotating the device in the solution 10 times while pushing against the vial wall. Swirl the brush vigorously to further release material. Discard the brush. Close the ThinPrep vial tightly. If the vial is not closed tightly, the sample will leak out during transport and will be lost.

The paintbrush-type brush (e.g., Cervex Brush) is used for collecting both ectocervical and endocervical cells at the same time. This brush has flexible plastic bristles, which are reported to cause less blood spotting after the examination. Introduce the brush into the vagina, and insert the central long bristles into the cervical os

Continued.

Obtaining Vaginal Smears and Cultures—cont'd

until the lateral bristles bend fully against the ectocervix. Maintain gentle pressure, and rotate the brush by rolling the handle between the thumb and forefinger three to five times to the left and right. Withdraw the brush, and transfer the sample to a glass slide with two single "paint" strokes. Apply first one side of the bristle, then turn the brush over, and paint the slide again in exactly the same area. Apply fixative, and label as the ectocervical and endocervical specimens.

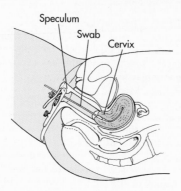

Speculum
Swab
Cervix

For the ThinPrep technology procedure, insert the central bristles of the broom into the endocervical canal deep enough to allow the shorter bristles to fully contact the ectocervix. Push gently, and rotate the broom clockwise **five** times. Rinse the broom into the solution vial by pushing the broom into the bottom of the vial 10 times, forcing the bristles apart. As a final step, swirl the broom vigorously to further release material. Discard the collection device. Close the ThinPrep vial tightly. If the vial is not closed tightly, the sample will leak out during transport and will be lost.

Gonococcal Culture Specimen

Immediately after the Pap smear is obtained, introduce a sterile cotton swab into the vagina, and insert it into the cervical os. Hold it in place for 10 to 30 seconds. Withdraw the swab, and spread the specimen in a large Z pattern over the culture medium, rotating the swab at the same time. Label the tube or plate, and follow agency routine for transporting and warming the specimen. If indicated, an anal culture can be obtained after the vaginal speculum has been removed. Insert a fresh, sterile cotton swab about 2.5 cm into the rectum, and rotate it in a full circle. Hold it in place for 10 to 30 seconds. Withdraw the swab, and prepare the specimen as described for the

Obtaining Vaginal Smears and Cultures—cont'd

vaginal culture. Gonococcal cultures are now used less frequently than the combined DNA probe for *Chlamydia* and gonorrhea.

DNA Probe for *Chlamydia* and Gonorrhea

This test involves the construction of a nucleic acid sequence (called a probe) that will match a sequence in the DNA or RNA of the target tissue. Results are rapid and sensitive. Use a Dacron swab (with a plastic or wire shaft) when collecting the specimen; wooden, cotton-tipped applicators may interfere with test results. Also be sure to check the expiration date so as not to use out-of-date materials. Insert the swab into the cervical os, and rotate the swab in the endocervical canal for 30 seconds to ensure adequate sampling and absorption by the swab. Avoid contact with the vaginal mucous membranes, which would contaminate the specimen. Remove the swab, and place it in the tube containing the specimen reagent.

Wet Mount and Potassium Hydroxide (KOH) Procedures

In a woman with vaginal discharge, these microscope examinations can demonstrate the presence of *Trichomonas vaginalis,* bacterial vaginosis, or candidiasis. For the wet mount, obtain a specimen of vaginal discharge using a swab. Smear the sample on a glass slide, and add a drop of normal saline solution. Place a coverslip on the slide, and view under the microscope. The presence of trichomonads indicates *T. vaginalis.* The presence of bacteria-filled epithelial cells (clue cells) indicates bacterial vaginosis. On a separate glass slide, place a specimen of vaginal discharge, apply a drop of aqueous 10% KOH, and put a coverslip in place. The presence of a fishy odor (the "whiff test") suggests bacterial vaginosis. The KOH dissolves epithelial cells and debris and facilitates visualization of the mycelia of a fungus. View under the microscope for the presence of mycelial fragments, hyphae, and budding yeast cells, which indicate candidiasis.

TECHNIQUE	FINDINGS

Internal Genitalia—Bimanual Examination—cont'd

Palpate cervix

Locate cervix with palmar surface of fingers, feel end, and run fingers around circumference to feel fornices.

■ *Size, shape, length*

EXPECTED: Consistent with speculum examination.

TECHNIQUE	FINDINGS
■ *Consistency*	**EXPECTED:** Firm in nonpregnant woman; softer in pregnant woman. **UNEXPECTED:** Nodules, hardness, or roughness.
■ *Position*	**EXPECTED:** In midline horizontal or pointing anteriorly or posteriorly. Protruding into vagina 1 to 3 cm. **UNEXPECTED:** Deviation to right or left. Protrusion into vagina greater than 1 to 3 cm.
■ *Mobility* Grasp cervix gently between fingers and move from side to side. Observe patient's facial expression.	**EXPECTED:** 1- to 2-cm movement in each direction. Minimal discomfort. **UNEXPECTED:** Pain on movement ("cervical motion tenderness").

Palpate uterus

■ *Location and position*
Place palmar surface of outside hand on abdominal midline, halfway between umbilicus and symphysis pubis, and place intravaginal fingers in anterior fornix. As shown in figure at right, slowly slide outside hand toward pubis while pressing down and forward with flat surface of fingers; at the same time, push inward and up with fingertips of intravaginal hand while pushing down on cervix with backs of fingers. If uterus is anteverted or anteflexed, you should feel fundus between fingers of two hands at level of pubis.

EXPECTED: In midline, horizontal, or pointing anteriorly or posteriorly. Protruding into vagina 1 to 3 cm.
UNEXPECTED: Deviation to right or left. Protrusion into vagina greater than 1 to 3 cm.

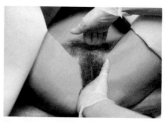

From Edge and Miller, 1994.

TECHNIQUE	FINDINGS

If uterus cannot be felt with this maneuver, place intravaginal fingers together in posterior fornix and outside hand immediately above symphysis pubis. Press firmly down with outside hand while pressing inward against cervix with intravaginal hand. If uterus is retroverted or retroflexed, you should feel fundus. If uterus cannot be felt with either of these maneuvers, move intravaginal fingers to each side of cervix, and while keeping contact with cervix, press inward and feel as far as possible. Slide fingers so they are on top and bottom of cervix and continue pressing in while moving fingers to feel as much of uterus as possible. (When uterus is in midposition, you will not be able to feel it with outside hand.)

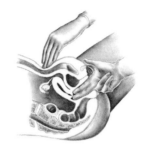

Anteverted

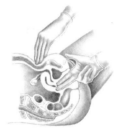

Anteflexed

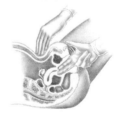

Retroverted

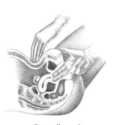

Retroflexed

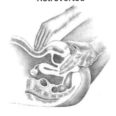

Midposition

TECHNIQUE	FINDINGS
■ *Size, shape, contour*	**EXPECTED:** Pear shaped and 5.5 to 8.0 cm long (larger in all dimensions in multiparous women). Contour rounded, and in nonpregnant women, walls firm and smooth. **UNEXPECTED:** Larger than expected or interrupted contour or smoothness.
■ *Mobility* Gently move uterus between intravaginal fingers and outside hand.	**EXPECTED:** Mobile in anteroposterior plane. **UNEXPECTED:** Fixed uterus or tenderness on movement.
Palpate ovaries	
Place fingers of outside hand on lower right quadrant. With intravaginal hand facing up, place both fingers in right lateral fornix. Press intravaginal fingers deeply in and up toward abdominal hand, while sweeping flat surface of fingers of outside hand deeply in and obliquely down toward symphysis pubis. Palpate entire area by firmly pressing outside hand and intravaginal fingers together. Repeat on left side.	
■ *Consistency*	**EXPECTED:** If palpable, ovaries should feel firm, smooth, slightly to moderately tender. **UNEXPECTED:** Marked tenderness or nodularity. Palpable fallopian tubes.

TECHNIQUE	FINDINGS
■ *Size*	**EXPECTED:** About 3 × 2 × 1 cm. **UNEXPECTED:** Enlargement.
■ *Shape*	**EXPECTED:** Ovoid.

Palpate adnexal areas

Use hand positions for palpating ovaries.	**EXPECTED:** Adnexae difficult to palpate. **UNEXPECTED:** Masses and tenderness. If adnexal masses are found, characterize by size, shape, location, consistency, tenderness.

Internal Genitalia—Rectovaginal Examination

Change gloves.

This examination may be uncomfortable for the patient. Assure her that although she may feel the urgency of a bowel movement, she will not have one. Ask her to breathe slowly and try to relax her sphincter, rectum, buttocks.

Insert index finger into vagina and middle finger into anus

To insert middle finger into anus, press against anus and ask patient to bear down. As she does, slip tip of finger into rectum just past sphincter.

Assess sphincter tone

Palpate area of anorectal junction and just above it. Ask patient to tighten and relax anal sphincter.	**EXPECTED:** Even sphincter tightening. **UNEXPECTED:** Extremely tight, lax, or absent sphincter.

TECHNIQUE	FINDINGS

Palpate anterior rectal wall and rectovaginal septum

Slide both fingers in as far as possible, then ask patient to bear down. Rotate rectal finger to explore anterior rectal wall and palpate rectovaginal septum.

EXPECTED: Smooth and uninterrupted. Uterine body and uterine fundus sometimes felt with retroflexed uterus.
UNEXPECTED: Masses, polyps, nodules, strictures, irregularities, tenderness.

Palpate posterior aspect of uterus

Place outside hand just above symphysis pubis and press firmly and deeply down, while positioning intravaginal finger in posterior vaginal fornix and pressing strongly upward against posterior side of cervix, as shown in figure at right. Palpate as much of posterior side of uterus as possible.

EXPECTED: Consistent with bimanual examination regarding location, position, size, shape, contour.
UNEXPECTED: Tenderness.

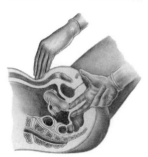

Palpate posterior rectal wall

As you withdraw fingers, rotate intrarectal finger to evaluate posterior rectal wall.

EXPECTED: Smooth and uninterrupted.
UNEXPECTED: Masses, polyps, nodules, strictures, irregularities, tenderness.

Note characteristics of feces when gloved finger removed

EXPECTED: Light to dark brown.
UNEXPECTED: Blood. Note color of any blood and prepare specimen for fecal occult blood testing (FOBT).

TECHNIQUE	FINDINGS

Wipe patient's perineum, using front-to-back stroke and clean tissue for each stroke

AIDS TO DIFFERENTIAL DIAGNOSIS

ABNORMALITY	DESCRIPTION
Premenstrual syndrome (PMS)	Edema, headache, weight gain, behavior disturbances such as irritability, nervousness, dysphoria, lack of coordination. Symptoms occur 5 to 7 days before menses, then subside.
Endometriosis	Pelvic pain, dysmenorrhea, heavy or prolonged menstrual flow.
Condyloma acuminatum (genital warts)	Warty lesions on labia, within vestibule, or in perianal region. Growths (generally whitish-pink to reddish-brown, discrete, soft) may occur singly or in clusters and may enlarge to cauliflower masses.
Herpes lesions	Small, red vesicles that may itch and usually are painful. Initial infection often extensive; recurrent infection normally a localized patch on vulva, perineum, vagina, or cervix.
Vaginal infections	Often vaginal discharge, possibly accompanied by urinary symptoms. Sometimes asymptomatic (see table on pp. 178-179).
Cervical carcinoma	Hard granular surface at or near cervical os. Lesion can evolve to form extensive, irregular, easily bleeding cauliflower growth.
Uterine bleeding	See table on p. 180.
Pelvic inflammatory disease (PID)	*Acute PID:* Very tender bilateral adnexal areas. *Chronic PID:* Bilateral tender, irregular, fairly fixed adnexal areas.

Differential Diagnosis of Vaginal Discharges and Infections

Condition	History	Physical Findings	Diagnostic Tests
Physiologic vaginitis	Increase in discharge; no foul odor, itching, or edema	Clear or mucoid discharge; pH < 4.5	Wet mount: up to 3-5 white blood cells (WBCs); epithelial cells
Bacterial vaginosis (Gardnerella vaginalis)	Foul-smelling discharge; complains of "fishy odor"	Homogeneous, thin, white or gray discharge; pH > 4.5	+ KOH "whiff" test; wet mount: + clue cells
Candida vulvovaginitis (Candida albicans)	Pruritic discharge, itching of labia; itching may extend to thighs	White, curdy discharge; pH 4.0-5.0; cervix may be red; may have erythema of perineum and thighs	KOH prep: mycelia, budding, branching yeast, pseudohyphae
Trichomoniasis (Trichomonas vaginalis)	Watery discharge; foul odor; dysuria and dyspareunia with severe infection	Profuse, frothy, greenish discharge; pH 5.0-6.6; red, friable cervix with petechiae ("strawberry" cervix)	Wet mount: round or pear-shaped protozoa, motile "gyrating" flagella
Gonorrhea (Neisseria gonorrhoeae)	Partner with sexually transmitted disease; often asymptomatic or may have symptoms of pelvic inflammatory disease	Purulent discharge from cervix; Skene/Bartholin gland inflammation; cervix and vulva may be inflamed	Gram stain, culture, DNA probe
Chlamydia (Chlamydia trachomatis)	Partner with nongonococcal urethritis; often asymptomatic; may complain of spotting after intercourse or urethritis	+/- purulent discharge; cervix may or may not be red or friable	DNA probe

Atrophic vaginitis	Dyspareunia; vaginal dryness; perimenopausal or postmenopausal	Pale, thin vaginal mucosa; pH > 4.5	Wet mount: folded, clumped epithelial cells
Allergic vaginitis	New bubble bath, soap, douche, or other hygiene products	Foul smell, erythema; pH < 4.5	Wet mount: WBCs
Foreign body	Red and swollen vulva; vaginal discharge; history of tampon, condom, or diaphragm use	Bloody or foul-smelling discharge	Wet mount: WBCs

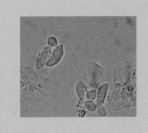

Trichomoniasis

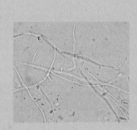

Candida vulvovaginitis

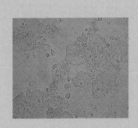

Bacterial vaginosis

Types of Uterine Bleeding and Associated Causes

Type	Common Causes
Midcycle spotting	Midcycle estradiol fluctuation associated with ovulation
Delayed menstruation with excessive bleeding	Anovulation or threatened abortion
Frequent bleeding	Chronic pelvic inflammatory disease, endometriosis, dysfunctional uterine bleeding (DUB), anovulation
Profuse menstrual bleeding	Endometrial polyps, DUB, adenomyosis, submucous leiomyomas, intrauterine device
Intermenstrual or irregular bleeding	Endometrial polyps, DUB, uterine or cervical cancer, oral contraceptives
Postmenopausal bleeding	Endometrial hyperplasia, estrogen therapy, endometrial cancer

Modified from Thompson et al, 1997.

PEDIATRIC VARIATIONS
EXAMINATION

TECHNIQUE	FINDINGS
Inspect external genitalia	
Examine infant using the frog-leg position.	**EXPECTED:** Genitalia of newborn reflects influence of maternal hormones. Labia majora and minora may be swollen, with labia minora often more prominent.
Inspect clitoris	
■ Size and length	**EXPECTED:** The clitoris of a term infant is usually covered by labia minora and may appear relatively large.

TECHNIQUE	FINDINGS

Inspect urethral meatus and vaginal opening

- *Inspect for discharge in infants and children*

EXPECTED: Mucoid whitish vaginal discharge is frequently seen during newborn period and sometimes as late as 4 weeks after birth. Discharge may be mixed with blood.
UNEXPECTED: Mucoid discharge from irritation by diapers or powder; any discharge in children.

Early Signs of Pregnancy

Following are physical signs that occur early in pregnancy. These signs, along with internal ballottement, palpation of fetal parts, and positive test results for urine or serum human chorionic gonadotropin, are probable indicators of pregnancy. They are considered "probable" because clinical conditions other than pregnancy may cause any one of them. Their occurrence together, however, creates a strong case for the presence of a pregnancy.

Sign	Finding	Aproximate Weeks of Gestation
Goodell	Softening of cervix	4-6
Hegar	Softening of uterine isthmus	6-8
McDonald	Easy flexing of fundus on cervix	7-8
Braun von Fernwald	Fullness and softening of fundus near site of implantation	7-8
Piskacek	Palpable lateral bulge or soft prominence of one uterine cornu	7-8
Chadwick	Bluish color of cervix, vagina, vulva	8-12

"Red Flags" for Sexual Abuse

The following signs and symptoms in children or adolescents should raise your suspicion for sexual abuse. Remember, however, that any sign or symptom by itself is of limited significance; it may be related to sexual abuse, or it may be from another cause altogether. This is an area in which good clinical judgment is imperative. Each sign or symptom must be considered in context with the particular child's health status, stage of growth and development, and entire history.

Medical Complaints and Findings

- Evidence of general physical abuse or neglect
- Evidence of trauma and/or scarring in genital, anal, and perianal areas
- Unusual changes in skin color or pigmentation in genital or anal area
- Presence of sexually transmitted disease (oral, anal, genital)
- Anorectal problems such as itching, bleeding, pain, fecal incontinence, poor anal sphincter tone, bowel habit dysfunction
- Genitourinary problems such as rash or sores in genital area, vaginal odor, pain (including abdominal pain), itching, bleeding, discharge, dysuria, hematuria, urinary tract infections, enuresis

Behavioral Manifestations

- Use of sexually provocative mannerisms, excessive masturbation, unusual or inappropriate sexual knowledge or experience
- Problems with school
- Dramatic weight changes or eating disturbances
- Depression
- Sleep problems or nightmares

Modified from Koop, 1988; McClain et al, 2000.

SAMPLE DOCUMENTATION

Subjective. A 45-year-old female with vaginal discharge and itching for past week. Has had yeast infections before. Completed course of antibiotics for sinusitis 2 days ago. Last menstrual period 2 weeks ago. Sexually active, one partner, mutually monogamous. No unusual vaginal bleeding. Does not douche.

Objective. *External:* Female hair distribution; no masses, lesions, or swelling. Urethral meatus intact without erythema or discharge. Perineum intact with healed episiotomy scar present. No lesions. *Internal:* Vaginal mucosa pink and moist with rugae present. No unusual odors. Profuse thick, white, curdy discharge. Cervix pink with horizontal slit midline; no lesions or discharge. *Bimanual:* Cervix smooth, firm, mobile. No cervical motion tenderness. Uterus midline, anteverted, firm, smooth, nontender; not enlarged. Ovaries not palpable. No adnexal tenderness. *Rectovaginal:* Septum intact. Sphincter tone intact; anal ring smooth and intact. No masses or tenderness.

Clinical and Reference Notes

15

Male Genitalia

EQUIPMENT

- Gloves
- Penlight

EXAMINATION

Have patient lying or standing to start examination.

TECHNIQUE	FINDINGS
Wear gloves on both hands	
Inspect pubic hair	
■ *Characteristics*	**EXPECTED:** Coarser than scalp hair.
■ *Distribution*	**EXPECTED:** Male hair distribution. Abundant in pubic region, continuing around scrotum to anal orifice, possibly continuing in narrowing midline to umbilicus. Penis without hair, scrotum with scant hair. **UNEXPECTED:** Alopecia.

TECHNIQUE	FINDINGS

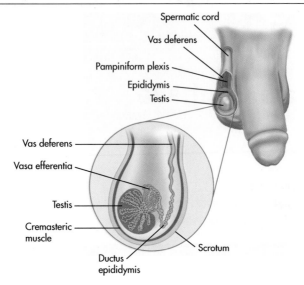

Inspect glans penis

- *Uncircumcised patient*
  Retract foreskin or ask patient to do so.

  EXPECTED: Dorsal vein apparent. Foreskin easily retracted. White, cheesy smegma visible over glans.
  UNEXPECTED: Tight foreskin (phimosis). Lesions or discharge.

- *Circumcised patient*

  EXPECTED: Dorsal vein apparent. Exposed glans erythematous and dry.
  UNEXPECTED: Lesions or discharge.

Examine external meatus of urethra (foreskin retracted in uncircumcised patient)

- *Shape*

  EXPECTED: Slitlike opening.
  UNEXPECTED: Pinpoint or round opening.

TECHNIQUE	FINDINGS
■ *Location*	**EXPECTED:** On ventral surface and only millimeters from tip of glans. **UNEXPECTED:** Any place other than tip of glans or along shaft of penis.
■ *Urethral orifice* Press glans between thumb and forefinger.	**EXPECTED:** Opening glistening and pink. **UNEXPECTED:** Bright erythema or discharge.
Palpate penis	**EXPECTED:** Soft (flaccid penis). **UNEXPECTED:** Tenderness, induration, or nodularity. Prolonged erection (priapism).
Strip urethra Firmly compress base of penis with thumb and forefinger; move toward glans.	**UNEXPECTED:** Discharge.
Inspect scrotum and ventral surface of penis	
■ *Color*	**EXPECTED:** Darker than body skin and often reddened in red-haired patients.
■ *Texture*	**EXPECTED:** Surface possibly coarse. Small lumps on scrotal skin (sebaceous or epidermoid cysts) that sometimes discharge oily material.
■ *Shape*	**EXPECTED:** Asymmetry. Thickness varying with temperature, age, emotional state. **UNEXPECTED:** Unusual thickening, often with pitting.

TECHNIQUE	FINDINGS

Palpate inguinal canal for direct or indirect hernia

With patient standing, ask him to bear down as if for bowel movement. While he strains, inspect area of inguinal canal and region of fossa ovalis. Ask patient to relax, and insert examining finger into lower part of scrotum and carry upward along vas deferens into inguinal canal, as shown in figure at right. Ask patient to cough. Repeat examination on opposite side.

EXPECTED: Presence of oval external ring.
UNEXPECTED: Feeling a viscus against examining finger with coughing. If hernia felt, note as indirect (felt within inguinal canal or even into scrotum) or direct (felt medial to external canal).

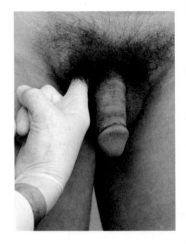

Palpate testes

Use thumb and first two fingers.

■ *Consistency*

EXPECTED: Smooth and rubbery. Sensitive to gentle compression.
UNEXPECTED: Tenderness or nodules. Total insensitivity to painful stimuli.

■ *Texture*

UNEXPECTED: Irregular texture.

TECHNIQUE	FINDINGS
■ *Size*	**UNEXPECTED:** Irregular size; asymmetry in size, less than 1 cm or greater than 5 cm.
■ *Descension*	**UNEXPECTED:** Cryptorchidism.
Palpate epididymides	**EXPECTED:** Smooth and discrete, with larger part cephalad.
	UNEXPECTED: Tenderness.
Palpate vas deferens	
Palpate from testicle to inguinal ring. Repeat with other testicle.	**EXPECTED:** Smooth and discrete.
	UNEXPECTED: Beaded or lumpy.
Palpate for inguinal lymph nodes	
Ask patient to lie supine, with knee slightly flexed on side of palpation.	**EXPECTED:** Nodes unable to be palpated.
	UNEXPECTED: Enlarged, tender, red or discolored, fixed, matted, inflamed, or warm nodes and increased vascularity.
Elicit cremasteric reflex bilaterally	
Stroke inner thigh with blunt instrument. Repeat with other thigh.	**EXPECTED:** Testicle and scrotum on stroked side rise.

AIDS TO DIFFERENTIAL DIAGNOSIS

ABNORMALITY	DESCRIPTION
Herpes	Superficial vesicles—located on glans, penile shaft, or base of penis—that are frequently quite painful. Often associated with inguinal lymphadenopathy and systemic symptoms (e.g., fever) in primary infection.
Hernia	See table on p. 190.

Distinguishing Characteristics of Hernias

	Indirect Inguinal	Direct Inguinal	Femoral
Incidence	Most common type of hernia; both sexes are affected; often patients are children and young males	Less common than indirect inguinal; occurs more often in males than females; more common in those older than 40 years	Least common type of hernia; occurs more often in females than males; rare in children
Occurrence	Through internal inguinal ring; can remain in canal, exit external ring, or pass into scrotum; may be bilateral	Through external inguinal ring; located in region of Hesselbach triangle; rarely enters scrotum	Through femoral ring, femoral canal, fossa ovalis
Presentation	Soft swelling in area of internal ring; pain on straining; hernia comes down canal and touches fingertip on examination	Bulge in area of Hesselbach triangle; usually painless; easily reduced; hernia bulges anteriorly, pushes against side of finger on examination	Right side presentation more common than left; pain may be severe; inguinal canal empty on examination

ABNORMALITY	DESCRIPTION
Hydrocele	Nontender, smooth, firm mass in scrotum. Transilluminates.
Varicocele	Abnormal tortuosity and dilated veins of pampiniform plexus within spermatic cord. Generally on left side and sometimes painful.
Epididymitis	Pain and possible erythema of overlying scrotum. Fever and white blood cells and bacteria in urine often accompany condition. In chronic form, epididymis feels firm and lumpy and may be slightly tender, and vasa deferentia may be beaded.
Priapism	Prolonged painful penile erection. May occur in patients with leukemia or sickle cell disease.
Hypospadias	Urethral meatus is located on ventral surface of glans, penile shaft, or perineal area.
Epispadias	Urethral meatus is located on dorsal surface of penile shaft.

PEDIATRIC VARIATIONS

EXAMINATION

TECHNIQUE	FINDINGS
Inspect glans penis	
■ *Uncircumcised patient* Retract foreskin.	**EXPECTED:** In children, foreskin is fully retractable by age 3 to 4 years. Before that age, forced retraction of foreskin may result in injury.

TECHNIQUE	FINDINGS
Palpate scrotum	
■ *Descension*	
Palpate testes in children to determine whether testes have descended.	**EXPECTED:** Bilaterally palpable; 1 cm. Considered descended if testis can be pushed into scrotum.
If any mass other than testicles or spermatic cord is palpated in scrotum, determine whether it is filled with fluid, gas, or solid material.	**UNEXPECTED:** If penlight transilluminates, most likely contains fluid (hydrocele). If no light transillumination, most likely a hernia.

SAMPLE DOCUMENTATION

Genitalia. Circumcised. Glans, penile shaft, contents of scrotal sac are intact without lesions or areas of induration. Urethral meatus patent on ventral surface at tip of glans. No discharge evident. Scrotal contents smooth without swelling, masses, or tenderness. Testes equal size. Inguinal areas are smooth; no masses or nodes palpable. Inguinal canals are free of masses, bulges. Cremasteric reflex elicited.

16

Anus, Rectum, and Prostate

EQUIPMENT

- Gloves
- Water-soluble lubricant
- Penlight
- Drapes
- Fecal occult blood testing materials

EXAMINATION

Have patient in knee-chest or left lateral position with hips and knees flexed, or standing with hips flexed and upper body supported by examining table. Drape patient appropriately.

TECHNIQUE	FINDINGS
Wear gloves on both hands	
Inspect and palpate sacrococcygeal and perianal area	
■ *Skin characteristics*	**EXPECTED:** Smooth and uninterrupted. **UNEXPECTED:** Lumps, rashes, tenderness, inflammation, excoriation, pilonidal dimpling, or tufts of hair.

TECHNIQUE	FINDINGS

Inspect anus

Spread patient's buttocks. Examine, using penlight or lamp if needed, with patient relaxed as well as with patient bearing down.

■ *Skin characteristics*

EXPECTED: Skin coarser and darker than on buttocks.
UNEXPECTED: Skin lesions, skin tags or warts, external or internal hemorrhoids, fissures and fistulas, rectal prolapse, or polyps. Describe any irregularities and locate using clock referents (12 o'clock ventral midline/6 o'clock dorsal midline).

Inspect, palpate, assess sphincter tone

Put water-soluble lubricant on index finger; press pad against anal opening, and ask patient to bear down to relax external sphincter. As relaxation occurs, slip tip of finger into anal canal, as shown in figure at right. (Assure patient that although he or she may feel the urgency of a bowel movement, it will not occur.) Ask patient to tighten external sphincter around finger.

EXPECTED: Even sphincter tightening.
UNEXPECTED: Patient discomfort. Lax or extremely tight sphincter, tenderness.

Deep external sphincter
Superficial external sphincter
Internal sphincter
Subcutaneous external sphincter
Levator ani muscle
Subcutaneous external sphincter

Palpate muscular anal ring

Rotate finger.

EXPECTED: Smooth, even with consistent pressure exerted.
UNEXPECTED: Nodules or other irregularities.

TECHNIQUE	FINDINGS

Palpate lateral and posterior rectal walls

Insert finger farther, and rotate to palpate lateral, then posterior, rectal walls. (If helpful, perform bidigital palpation with thumb and index finger by lightly pressing thumb against perianal tissue and bringing index finger toward thumb.)

EXPECTED: Smooth, even, uninterrupted.
UNEXPECTED: Nodules, masses, polyps, tenderness, or irregularities. (Internal hemorrhoids not ordinarily felt unless thrombosed.)

Males: Palpate posterior surface of prostate gland through anterior rectal wall

Rotate finger and palpate anterior rectal wall and posterior surface of prostate gland. (Alert patient that he may feel urge to urinate but will not.)

- *Consistency and characteristics of anterior rectal wall*

EXPECTED: Smooth, even, uninterrupted.
UNEXPECTED: Nodules, masses, polyps, tenderness, or irregularities.

- *Consistency, contour, characteristics of prostate*

EXPECTED: Surface firm and smooth, lateral lobes symmetric, median sulcus palpable, seminal vesicles not palpable.
UNEXPECTED: Rubberiness, bogginess, fluctuant softness, stony hard nodularity, tenderness, obliterated sulcus, or palpable seminal vesicles.

- *Mobility of prostate gland*

EXPECTED: Slightly movable.

- *Size of prostate gland*

EXPECTED: 4 cm diameter with less than 1 cm protruding into rectum.
UNEXPECTED: Protrusion greater than 1 cm (note distance of protrusion).

TECHNIQUE	FINDINGS
	UNEXPECTED: Discharge that appears at urethral meatus (collect specimen for microscopic examination).

Females: Palpate uterus through anterior rectal wall

Attempt to palpate uterus and cervix through anterior rectal wall.	
■ *Position*	**EXPECTED:** Midline, retroflexed or retroverted.
	UNEXPECTED: Deviation to right or left.
■ *Surface characteristics*	**EXPECTED:** Smooth.
	UNEXPECTED: Irregular.

Have patient bear down, and palpate deeper

Ask patient to bear down while you reach farther into rectum. *Females:* Explore in cul-de-sac. *Males:* Explore above prostate.	**UNEXPECTED:** Tenderness of peritoneal area or nodules.

Withdraw finger, and examine fecal material

■ *Color and consistency*	**EXPECTED:** Soft and brown.
	UNEXPECTED: Blood; pus; or light-tan, gray, or tarry-black stool. Test any fecal material for blood using chemical fecal occult blood testing (FOBT) procedure.

AIDS TO DIFFERENTIAL DIAGNOSIS

ABNORMALITY	DESCRIPTION
Perianal and perirectal abscesses	Pain and tenderness in anal area, usually accompanied by a fever.
Enterobiasis infestation in children	Intense perianal itching, especially at night.

ABNORMALITY	DESCRIPTION
Anorectal fissure and fistula	*Fissure:* Pain, itching, or bleeding, with spastic internal sphincter. *Fistula:* Elevated, red, granular tissue at external opening, possibly with serosanguinous or purulent drainage on compression of the area.
Hemorrhoids	*External:* Itching and bleeding with defecation. Thrombosed hemorrhoids appear as blue, shiny masses at anus. *Internal:* Bleeding with or without defecation. Do not cause discomfort unless thrombosed, prolapsed, or infected.
Rectal carcinoma	Generally asymptomatic.
Prostatic carcinoma	On rectal examination, a hard irregular nodule may be palpable. Prostate feels asymmetric and median sulcus is obliterated in advanced carcinoma.
Benign prostatic hypertrophy	Hesitancy on urination, decreased force and caliber of stream, dribbling, incomplete emptying of bladder, nocturia, dysuria.

PEDIATRIC VARIATIONS
EXAMINATION

TECHNIQUE	FINDINGS
Inspect perianal area	**UNEXPECTED:** Parental complaints of infant's or child's irritability at night or evidence that child has itching in perianal area may indicate presence of parasites such as round worms or pinworms. Specimen collection and microscopic examination are necessary to confirm findings.

Subjective. A 57-year-old male complains of nighttime urination for the past several months, at least twice per night. Restricts fluid intake after 8 PM. Notices difficulty in starting stream. No pain or bleeding on urination. No change in caliber of stream. Denies change in bowel habits or stool characteristics. No history of prostatitis or enlarged prostate.

Objective. Perianal area intact without lesions or visible hemorrhoids. An external skin tag is visible in the 6 o'clock position. No fissures or fistulas. Sphincter tightens evenly. Prostate is symmetric, smooth, boggy, with 1-cm protrusion into rectum. Medial sulcus present. Nontender, no nodules. Rectal walls free of masses. Moderate amount of soft stool present; occult blood test result negative.

17

Musculoskeletal System

EQUIPMENT

- Goniometer
- Skin-marking pencil
- Reflex hammer
- Tape measure

EXAMINATION

Begin examination as patient enters rooms, observing gait and posture. During examination, note ease of movement when patient walks, sits, rises, takes off garments, responds to directions.

TECHNIQUE	FINDINGS

Posture and General Guidelines

Inspect skeleton and extremities, comparing sides

Inspect anterior, posterior, lateral aspects of posture; ability to stand erect; body parts; extremities.

- *Size, alignment, contour, symmetry*

    Measure extremities when lack of symmetry is noted in length or circumference

EXPECTED: Bilateral symmetry of length, circumference, alignment, position and number of skin folds; symmetric body parts; and aligned extremities.

199

TECHNIQUE	FINDINGS

UNEXPECTED: Gross deformity, lordosis, kyphosis, scoliosis, bony enlargement.

Inspect skin and subcutaneous tissues over muscles, cartilage, bones, joints

UNEXPECTED: Discoloration, swelling, or masses.

Inspect muscles, and compare sides

- *Size and symmetry*

EXPECTED: Approximately symmetric bilateral muscle size.
UNEXPECTED: Gross hypertrophy or atrophy, fasciculations, or spasms.

Palpate all bones, joints, surrounding muscles (palpate inflamed joints last)

- *Muscle tone*

EXPECTED: Firm.
UNEXPECTED: Hard or doughy, spasticity.

- *Characteristics*

UNEXPECTED: Heat, tenderness, swelling, fluctuation of a joint, synovial thickening, crepitus, resistance to pressure, or discomfort to pressure on bones and joints.

Test each major joint and related muscle groups for active and passive range of motion, and compare sides

Ask patient to move each joint through range of motion (see instructions for specific joints and muscles in individual sections that follow), then ask patient to relax as you passively move same joints until end of range is felt.

EXPECTED: Passive range of motion often exceeds active range of motion by 5 degrees. Range of motion with passive and active maneuvers should be equal between contralateral joints.

TECHNIQUE	FINDINGS

UNEXPECTED: Pain, limitation of motion, spastic movement, joint instability, deformity, contracture, discrepancies greater than 5 degrees between active and passive range of motion. when increase or limitation in range of motion is found, measure angles of greatest flexion and extension with goniometer, as shown in figure below, and compare with values as described for specific joints in individual sections.

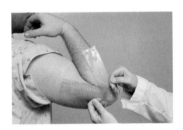

Muscle Strength Assessment

Muscle Function Level	Grade
No evidence of contractility	0
Slight contractility, no movement	1
Full range of motion, gravity eliminated*	2
Full range of motion against gravity	3
Full range of motion against gravity, some resistance	4
Full range of motion against gravity, full resistance	5

From Jacobson, 1998.
*Passive movement.

TECHNIQUE   FINDINGS

Test major muscle groups for strength, and compare contralateral
sides

For each muscle group, ask
patient to contract a muscle
by flexing or extending a
joint and to resist as you apply opposing force. Compare
bilaterally.

EXPECTED: Bilaterally symmetric with full resistance to
opposition.
UNEXPECTED: Inability to
produce full resistance. grade
muscular strength according to
table on p. 201.

Temporomandibular Joint

Palpate joint space for clicking, popping, pain

Locate temporomandibular
joints with fingertips placed
just anterior to tragus of each
ear, as shown in figure at
right. Ask patient to open
mouth and allow fingertips
to slip into joint space.
Gently palpate.

EXPECTED: Audible or palpable snapping or clicking may be
noted.
UNEXPECTED: Pain, crepitus,
locking, or popping.

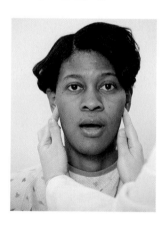

Test range of motion

Ask patient to:

■ *Open and close mouth*

EXPECTED: Opens 3 to 6 cm
between upper and lower teeth.

■ *Move jaw laterally to each side*

EXPECTED: Mandible moves 1
to 2 cm in each direction.

■ *Protrude and retract jaw*

EXPECTED: Both protrusion
and retraction possible.

TECHNIQUE	FINDINGS

Test strength of temporalis and masseter muscles with patient's teeth clenched

| Ask patient to clench teeth while you palpate contracted muscles and apply opposing force. (This also tests cranial nerve V motor function.) | **EXPECTED:** Bilaterally symmetric with full resistance to opposition.
UNEXPECTED: Inability to produce full resistance. |

Cervical Spine

Inspect neck from anterior and posterior positions

| ■ *Alignment* | **EXPECTED:** Cervical spine straight, with head erect and in approximate alignment. |
| ■ *Symmetry of skinfolds* | **UNEXPECTED:** Asymmetric skinfolds. |

Palpate posterior neck; cervical spine; and paravertebral, trapezius, and sternocleidomastoid muscles

| | **EXPECTED:** Good muscle tone, symmetry in size.
UNEXPECTED: Palpable tenderness or muscle spasm. |

Test range of motion

■ *Forward flexion* Bend head forward, chin to chest.	**EXPECTED:** 45-degree flexion.
■ *Hyperextension* Bend head backward, chin toward ceiling.	**EXPECTED:** 45-degree hyperextension.
■ *Lateral bending* Bend head to each side, ear to each shoulder.	**EXPECTED:** 40-degree lateral bending.
■ *Rotation* Turn head to each side, chin to shoulder.	**EXPECTED:** 70-degree rotation.

TECHNIQUE	FINDINGS

Test strength of sternocleidomastoid and trapezius muscles

Ask patient to maintain each of the previous positions while you apply opposing force. (Cranial nerve XI is also tested with rotation.)

EXPECTED: Bilaterally symmetric strength with full resistance to opposition.
UNEXPECTED: Inability to produce full resistance.

Thoracic and Lumbar Spine

Inspect spine for alignment

Note major landmarks of back—each spinal process of vertebrae (C7 and T1 usually most prominent), scapulae, iliac crests, paravertebral muscles.

EXPECTED: Head positioned directly over gluteal cleft, vertebrae straight (as indicated by symmetric shoulder, scapular, and iliac crest heights), curves of cervical and lumbar spines concave, curve of thoracic spine convex, and knees and feet aligned with trunk and pointing directly forward.
UNEXPECTED: Lordosis, kyphosis, scoliosis, or sharp angular deformity (gibbus).

Palpate spinal processes and paravertebral muscles

Ask patient to stand erect.

UNEXPECTED: Muscle spasm or spinal tenderness.

Percuss for spinal tenderness

Patient is still standing erect. First tap each spinal process with one finger, then rap each side of spine along paravertebral muscles with ulnar aspect of fist.

UNEXPECTED: Muscle spasm or spinal tenderness.

TECHNIQUE	FINDINGS

Test range of motion and curvature

Ask patient to perform following movements (mark each spinal process with skin pencil if unexpected curvature suspected):

■ *Forward flexion*
Bend forward at waist and try to touch toes. Observe patient from behind to check curvature.

EXPECTED: 75- to 90-degree flexion; back remains symmetrically flat as concave curve of lumbar spine becomes convex with forward flexion.
UNEXPECTED: Lateral curvature or rib hump.

■ *Hyperextension*
Bend back at waist as far as possible.

EXPECTED: 30-degree hyperextension with reversal of lumbar curve.

■ *Lateral bending*
Bend to each side as far as possible.

EXPECTED: 35-degree lateral bending on each side.

■ *Rotation*
Swing upper trunk from waist in circular motion, front to side to back to side, while you stabilize pelvis.

EXPECTED: 30-degree rotation forward and backward.

Test for lumbar nerve root irritation or disk herniation at L4, L5, or S1 levels (patient supine with neck slightly flexed)

■ *Straight leg raising test*
Ask patient to raise leg with knee extended. Repeat with other leg.

EXPECTED: No pain below knee with leg raising.
UNEXPECTED: Unable to raise leg more than 30 degrees without pain. flexion of knee often eliminates pain with leg raising. crossover pain in affected leg.

TECHNIQUE   FINDINGS

- *Bragard stretch test*
  Hold patient's lower leg with
  knee extended, and raise it
  slowly until pain is felt.
  Lower leg slightly, briskly
  dorsiflex foot, and internally
  rotate hip.

UNEXPECTED: Pain when leg
is raised less than 70 degrees;
aggravated by dorsiflexion and
internal rotation of hip.

Shoulders

Inspect shoulders, shoulder girdle, clavicles and scapulae, area
muscles

- *Size and contour*

EXPECTED: All shoulder structures symmetric in size and
contour.
UNEXPECTED: Asymmetry,
hollows in rounding contour, or
winged scapula.

Palpate sternoclavicular and acromioclavicular joints, clavicle,
scapulae, coracoid process, greater trochanter of humerus, biceps
groove, area muscles

EXPECTED: No tenderness or
masses, bilateral symmetry.
UNEXPECTED: Pain, tenderness, mass.

Test range of motion

Ask patient to perform fol-
lowing movements:
- *Shoulder shrug*
- *Forward flexion*
  Raise both arms forward and
  straight up over head.
- *Hyperextension*
  Extend and stretch both arms
  behind back.
- *Abduction*
  Lift both arms laterally and
  straight up over head.

EXPECTED: Symmetric rising.

EXPECTED: 180-degree forward flexion.

EXPECTED: 50-degree hyperextension.

EXPECTED: 180-degree abduction.

TECHNIQUE	FINDINGS

- *Adduction*
  Swing each arm across front of body.

  EXPECTED: 50-degree adduction.

- *Internal rotation*
  Place both arms behind hips, elbows out.

  EXPECTED: 90-degree internal rotation.

- *External*
  Place both arms behind head, elbows out.

  EXPECTED: 90-degree external rotation.

Test shoulder girdle muscle strength

Ask patient to maintain following positions while you apply opposing force:

- *Shrugged shoulders*
  (This also tests cranial nerve XI.)

  EXPECTED: Bilaterally symmetric with full resistance to opposition.
  UNEXPECTED: Inability to produce full resistance.

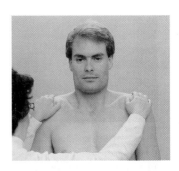

- *Forward flexion*

  EXPECTED: Bilaterally symmetric with full resistance to opposition.
  UNEXPECTED: Inability to produce full resistance.

TECHNIQUE	FINDINGS
■ *Abduction*	**EXPECTED:** Bilaterally symmetric with full resistance to opposition. **UNEXPECTED:** Inability to produce full resistance.

Elbows

Inspect elbows in flexed and extended positions

■ *Contour*	**UNEXPECTED:** Subcutaneous nodules along pressure points of extensor surface of ulna.
■ *Carrying angle* Inspect with arm passively extended, palm forward.	**EXPECTED:** Usually 5 to 15 degrees laterally. **UNEXPECTED:** Lateral angle exceeding 15 degrees (cubitus valgus) or a medial carrying angle (cubitus varus).

Palpate extensor surface of ulna, olecranon process, medial and lateral epicondyles of humerus, groove on each side of olecranon process

Palpate with patient's elbow flexed at 70 degrees.	**UNEXPECTED:** Boggy, soft, or fluctuant swelling; point tenderness at lateral epicondyle or along grooves of olecranon process and epicondyles.

Test range of motion

Ask patient to perform following movements:

■ *Flexion and extension* Bend and straighten elbow.	**EXPECTED:** 160-degree flexion from full extension at 0 degrees.
■ *Pronation and supination* With elbow flexed at right angle, rotate hand from palm side down to palm side up.	**EXPECTED:** 90-degree pronation and 90-degree supination. **UNEXPECTED:** Increased pain with pronation and supination of elbow.

TECHNIQUE	FINDINGS

Test muscle strength

Ask patient to maintain flexion and extension, as well as
pronation and supination,
while you apply opposing
force.

EXPECTED: Bilaterally symmetric with full resistance to
opposition.
UNEXPECTED: Inability to
produce full resistance.

Hands and Wrists

Inspect dorsum and palm of each hand

■ *Characteristics and contour*

EXPECTED: Palmar and phalangeal creases, palmar surfaces
with central depression with
prominent, rounded mound on
thumb side (thenar eminence)
and less prominent hypothenar
eminence on little-finger side.

■ *Position*

EXPECTED: Fingers able to
fully extend and aligned with
forearm when in close approxi-
mation to each other.
UNEXPECTED: Deviation of
fingers to ulnar side or swan-
neck or boutonnière deformities.

■ *Shape*

EXPECTED: Lateral finger surfaces gradually tapered from
proximal to distal aspects.
UNEXPECTED: Spindle-shaped
fingers, bony overgrowths at
phalangeal joints.

TECHNIQUE	FINDINGS

Palpate each joint in hand and wrist

Palpate interphalangeal joints with thumb and index finger, as shown in figure at right; metacarpophalangeal joints with both thumbs, as shown in figure below, left; and wrist and radiocarpal groove with thumbs on dorsal surface and fingers on palmar aspect of wrist, as shown in figure below, right.

EXPECTED: Joint surfaces smooth.
UNEXPECTED: Nodules, swelling, bogginess, tenderness, or ganglion.

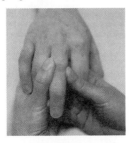

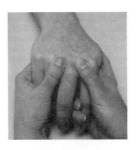

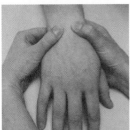

Assess integrity of median nerve

■ *Tinel sign*
Strike median nerve where it passes through carpal tunnel with index or middle finger.

UNEXPECTED: Tingling sensation radiating from wrist to hand along median nerve.

■ *Thumb abduction test*
Apply downward pressure on thumb as patient holds thumb perpendicular to hand, palm side up.

EXPECTED: Full resistance to pressure.
UNEXPECTED: Inability to produce full resistance.

TECHNIQUE	FINDINGS

■ *Phalen test*
Have patient hold both wrists in fully palmar-flexed position with dorsal surfaces pressed together for 1 minute.

UNEXPECTED: Numbness, paresthesia in distribution of median nerve.

■ *Katz hand diagram*
Have patient mark specific locations of pain, numbness, tingling in hands and arms on diagram.

UNEXPECTED: Pain, numbness, tingling in pattern shown in figure on p. 212.

Test range of motion

Ask patient to perform following movements:

■ *Metacarpophalangeal flexion and hyperextension*
Bend fingers forward at metacarpophalangeal joint, then stretch fingers up and back at knuckle.

EXPECTED: 90-degree metacarpophalangeal flexion and as much as 20-degree hyperextension.

■ *Thumb opposition*
Touch thumb to each fingertip and to base of little finger, then make a fist.

EXPECTED: Able to perform all movements.

■ *Finger abduction and adduction*
Spread fingers apart, and then touch them together.

EXPECTED: Both movements possible.

■ *Wrist extension and hyperextension*
Bend hand at wrist up and down.

EXPECTED: 90-degree flexion and 70-degree hyperextension.

■ *Radial and ulnar motion*
With palm side down, turn each hand to right and left.

EXPECTED: 20-degree radial motion and 55-degree ulnar motion.

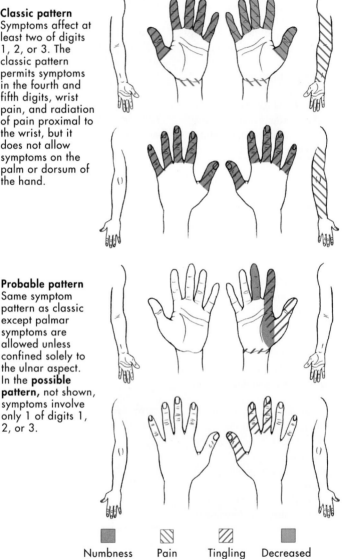

Classic pattern
Symptoms affect at least two of digits 1, 2, or 3. The classic pattern permits symptoms in the fourth and fifth digits, wrist pain, and radiation of pain proximal to the wrist, but it does not allow symptoms on the palm or dorsum of the hand.

Probable pattern
Same symptom pattern as classic except palmar symptoms are allowed unless confined solely to the ulnar aspect. In the **possible pattern**, not shown, symptoms involve only 1 of digits 1, 2, or 3.

Numbness   Pain   Tingling   Decreased sensation

Redrawn from D'Arcy and McGee, 2000.

TECHNIQUE	FINDINGS

Test muscle strength

Ask patient to perform following movements:

- *Wrist extension and hyperextension*
  Maintain wrist flexion while you apply opposing force.

EXPECTED: Bilaterally symmetric with full resistance to opposition.
UNEXPECTED: Inability to produce full resistance.

- *Hand strength*
  Grip two of your fingers tightly.

EXPECTED: Firm, sustained grip.
UNEXPECTED: Weakness or pain.

Hips

Inspect hips for symmetry and level of gluteal folds

With patient standing, inspect anteriorly and posteriorly, using major landmarks of iliac crest and greater trochanter of femur.

UNEXPECTED: Asymmetry in iliac crest height, size of buttocks, or number and level of gluteal folds.

Palpate hips and pelvis

Have patient lie supine.

UNEXPECTED: Instability, tenderness, or crepitus.

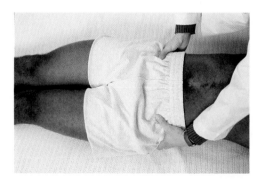

TECHNIQUE	FINDINGS

Test range of motion

While in position indicated, patient should perform following movements:

- *Flexion, knee extended*
  With patient supine, raise leg over body.

  EXPECTED: Up to 90-degree flexion.

- *Hyperextension*
  While standing or prone, swing straightened leg behind body without arching the back.

  EXPECTED: Up to 30-degree hyperextension.

- *Flexion, knee flexed*
  While supine, raise one knee to chest while keeping other leg straight.

  EXPECTED: 120-degree flexion.

- *Abduction and adduction*
  While supine, swing leg laterally and medially with knee straight. During adduction movement, lift patient's opposite leg to permit examined leg full movement.

  EXPECTED: Some degree of both abduction and adduction.

- *Internal rotation*
  While supine, flex knee and rotate leg inward toward other leg.

  EXPECTED: 40-degree internal rotation.

- *External rotation*
  While supine, place lateral aspect of foot on knee of other leg. Move flexed leg toward table.

  EXPECTED: 45-degree external rotation.

Test muscle strength

- *Knee in flexion and extension*
  Ask patient to maintain flexion of hip with knee in flexion and then extension while applying opposing force.

  EXPECTED: Bilaterally symmetric with full resistance to opposition.

TECHNIQUE	FINDINGS

| | **UNEXPECTED:** Inability to produce full resistance |
| ■ *Resistance to uncrossing legs while seated.* | **EXPECTED:** Bilaterally symmetric with full resistance to opposition. |

Perform Thomas test to inspect for flexion contractures

While supine, patient should fully extend one leg flat on examining table and flex other leg with knee to chest.	**EXPECTED:** Patient able to keep extended leg flat on table.
	UNEXPECTED: Extended leg lifts off table.

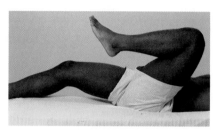

Perform Trendelenburg test to inspect for weak hip abductor muscles

Ask patient to stand and balance first on one foot, then on other. Observe from behind.	**UNEXPECTED:** Asymmetry or change in level of iliac crests.

Legs and Knees

Inspect knees and popliteal spaces, flexed and extended

Note major landmarks—tibial tuberosity, medial and lateral tibial condyles, medial and lateral epicondyles of femur, adductor tubercle of femur, patella.	**EXPECTED:** Natural concavities on anterior aspect, on each side, above patella.
	UNEXPECTED: Usual indentation above patella is convex rather than concave.

TECHNIQUE	FINDINGS
Observe lower leg alignment	**EXPECTED:** Angle between femur and tibia less than 15 degrees. Bowlegs common until 18 months of age; knock knees common between 2 and 4 years. **UNEXPECTED:** Knock knees (genu valgum), bowlegs (genu varum), excessive hyperextension of knee with weight bearing (genu recurvatum).
Palpate popliteal space	**UNEXPECTED:** Swelling or tenderness.
Palpate tibiofemoral joint space Identify patella, suprapatellar pouch, infrapatellar fat pad.	**EXPECTED:** Smooth and firm. **UNEXPECTED:** Tenderness, bogginess, nodules, or crepitus.
Test range of motion ■ *Flexion* Ask patient to bend each knee.	**EXPECTED:** 130-degree flexion.
■ *Extension* Ask patient to straighten leg and stretch it.	**EXPECTED:** Full extension and up to 15-degree hyperextension.
Test muscle strength ■ *Flexion and extension* Ask patient to maintain flexion and extension while you apply opposing force.	**EXPECTED:** Bilaterally symmetric with full resistance to opposition. **UNEXPECTED:** Inability to produce full resistance.

TECHNIQUE   FINDINGS

Additional Techniques for Knees

Perform ballottement procedure to determine presence of excess fluid or effusion in knee

With knee extended, apply downward pressure on supra-patellar pouch with thumb and finger of one hand, then push patella sharply downward against femur with fingers of other hand, as shown at right. Suddenly release pressure on patella, while keeping fingers lightly on knee.

UNEXPECTED: A tapping or clicking is sensed when patella is pushed against femur. Patella then floats out as if a fluid wave is pushing it.

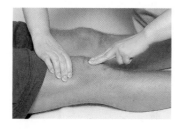

Test for bulge sign to determine presence of excess fluid in knee

With knee extended, milk medial aspect of knee upward two or three times, as shown in top figure at right, then tap lateral side of patella, as shown in bottom figure at right.

UNEXPECTED: Bulge of returning fluid to hollow area medial to patella.

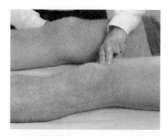

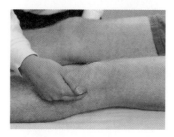

TECHNIQUE	FINDINGS

Perform McMurray test to detect torn meniscus

Ask patient to lie supine and flex one knee completely with foot flat on table near buttocks. Maintain that flexion with your thumb and index finger, while stabilizing knee. Hold heel with other hand; rotate foot and lower leg to lateral position. Extend knee to 90-degree angle. Return knee to full flexion, then repeat procedure rotating foot and lower leg.

UNEXPECTED: Palpable or audible click or limited extension of knee with either lateral or medial movements.

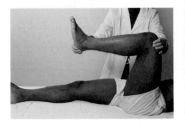

Perform drawer test to identify anteroposterior instability of cruciate ligaments

Ask patient, while supine, to flex knee 45 to 90 degrees, placing foot flat on table. Place both hands on lower leg with thumbs on ridge of anterior tibia near tibial tuberosity. Pull tibia, sliding it forward of femur. Then push tibia backwards.

UNEXPECTED: Anterior or posterior movement greater than 5 mm.

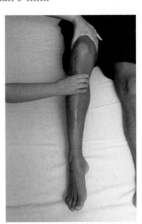

TECHNIQUE	FINDINGS

Perform varus valgus stress test to identify mediolateral instability of knee

Ask patient to lie supine and extend knee. While you stabilize femur with one hand and hold ankle with other, apply varus force (toward midline) and internal rotation. Then apply valgus force (away from midline) and external rotation. Repeat with knee flexed to 30 degrees.

UNEXPECTED: Excessive laxity, medial or lateral movement.

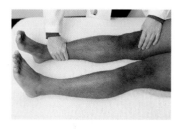

Perform Apley test to detect torn meniscus

Ask patient to lie prone and flex knee to 90 degrees. Place hand on heel of foot and press firmly, opposing tibia to femur. Carefully rotate lower leg externally and internally. Do not cause excess pain.

UNEXPECTED: Clicks, locking, or pain.

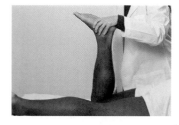

Feet and Ankles

Inspect during weight bearing (standing and walking) and non–weight bearing

Note major landmarks—medial malleolus, lateral malleolus, Achilles tendon.

- *Characteristics*

EXPECTED: Smooth and rounded malleolar prominence, prominent heels, prominent metatarsophalangeal joints.
UNEXPECTED: Calluses and corns.

TECHNIQUE	FINDINGS
■ *Alignment*	**EXPECTED:** Feet aligned with tibias and weight bearing on foot midline. **UNEXPECTED:** In-toeing (pes varus), out-toeing (pes valgus), deviations in forefoot alignment (metatarsus varus or metatarsus valgus), heel pronation, or pain.
■ *Contour*	**EXPECTED:** Longitudinal arch that may flatten with weight bearing. Foot flat when not bearing weight (pes planus) and high instep (pes cavus) are common variations. **UNEXPECTED:** Pain with pes planus.
■ *Toes*	**EXPECTED:** Toes on each foot straight forward, flat, in alignment. **UNEXPECTED:** Hammer toe; claw toe; mallet toe; hallux valgus; bunions; or heat, redness, swelling, tenderness of metatarsophalangeal joint of great toe (possibly with draining tophus).

Palpate Achilles tendon and each metatarsal joint

Using thumb and fingers of both hands, compress forefoot, palpating each metatarsophalangeal joint.	**EXPECTED:** No tenderness or masses, bilateral symmetry. **UNEXPECTED:** Pain, masses, thickened Achilles tendon.

Test range of motion

Ask patient to sit, then perform following movements:
■ *Dorsiflexion*
Point foot toward ceiling.

EXPECTED: 20-degree dorsiflexion.

TECHNIQUE	FINDINGS

- *Plantar flexion*
  Point foot toward floor.

  EXPECTED: 45-degree plantar flexion.

- *Inversion and eversion*
  Bend foot at ankle, then turn sole of foot toward and away from other foot.

  EXPECTED: 30-degree inversion and 20-degree eversion.

- *Abduction and adduction*
  Rotate ankle, turning away from and then toward other foot (while you stabilize leg).

  EXPECTED: 10-degree abduction and 20-degree adduction.

- *Flexion and extension*
  Bend and straighten toes.

  EXPECTED: Some flexion and extension, especially of great toes.

Test strength of ankle muscles

Ask patient to maintain dorsiflexion and plantar flexion while you apply opposing force.

EXPECTED: Bilaterally symmetric with full resistance to opposition.
UNEXPECTED: Inability to produce full resistance.

AIDS TO DIFFERENTIAL DIAGNOSIS

ABNORMALITY	DESCRIPTION
Carpal tunnel syndrome	Numbness, burning, tingling in hands, often occurring at night but also elicited by rotational movement of wrist. Pain in arms. Can result in weakness of hand and flattening of thenar eminence of palm.
Gout	Red, hot, swollen joint (classically proximal phalanx of great toe, although other joints of wrist, hands, ankles, knees are sometimes affected); exquisite pain; limited range of motion; tophi; and mild fever.

ABNORMALITY	DESCRIPTION
Lumbar disk herniation	Lower back pain with radiation to buttocks and posterior thigh or down leg in distribution of nerve root dermatome (see pp. 236-237), spasm or tenderness over paraspinal muscles, muscle weakness, paresthesia.
Bursitis	Motion limitation caused by swelling, pain on movement, point tenderness, erythema, warmth; commonly occurs in shoulder, elbow, hip, knee.
Osteoarthritis	See table on p. 223.
Rheumatoid arthritis	See table on p. 223.
Sprain	Pain, marked swelling, hemorrhage, loss of function associated with stretching or tearing of a joint ligament.
Fracture	Deformity, edema, pain, loss of function, color changes, paresthesia.
Tenosynovitis	Point tenderness; edema; pain with movement; and weakness, commonly of shoulder, knee, heel, wrist.
Scoliosis	Uneven shoulder and hip levels, rib hump, flank asymmetry on forward flexion. Lateral curvature of spine resulting from leg length discrepancy also possible.
Osteoporosis	Height loss, bent spine, appearance of sinking into hips—most often in postmenopausal women. Usual presenting symptom is acute, painful fracture, most commonly of hip, vertebra, or wrist.

Differential Diagnosis of Arthritis

Signs and Symptoms	Osteoarthritis	Rheumatoid Arthritis
Onset	Insidious	Gradual or sudden (24-48 hours)
Duration of stiffness	Few minutes, localized, but short "gelling" after prolonged rest	Often hours, most pronounced after rest
Pain	On motion, with prolonged activity, relieved by rest	Even at rest, may disturb sleep
Weakness	Usually localized and not severe	Often pronounced, out of proportion with muscle atrophy
Fatigue	Unusual	Often severe, with onset 4 to 5 hours after rising
Emotional depression and lability	Unusual	Common, coincides with fatigue and disease activity, often relieved if in remission
Tenderness localized over afflicted joint	Common	Almost always; most sensitive indicator of inflammation
Swelling	Effusion common, little synovial reaction, swelling rare	Fusiform soft tissue enlargement, effusion common, synovial proliferation and thickening
Heat, erythema	Unusual	Sometimes present
Crepitus, crackling	Coarse to medium on motion	Medium to fine
Joint enlargement	Mild with firm consistency	Moderate to severe

Modified from McCarty, 1993.

PEDIATRIC VARIATIONS

EXAMINATION

Musculoskeletal findings and motor development in infants, children, and adolescents change as they grow. For a complete description of age-specific anticipated pediatric findings, see Chapter 21.

Sports Participation Screening Examination for Children and Adolescents

- Observe posture and general muscle contour bilaterally.
- Observe gait.
- Ask patient to walk on tiptoes and heels.
- Observe patient hop on each foot.
- Ask patient to duck walk four steps with knees completely bent.
- Inspect spine for curvature and lumbar extension, fingers touching toes with knees straight.
- Palpate shoulder and clavicle for dislocation.
- Check following for range of motion—neck, shoulder, elbow, forearm, hands, fingers, hips.
- Test knee ligaments for drawer sign.

SAMPLE DOCUMENTATION

Subjective. A 13-year-old female referred by school nurse because of uneven shoulder and hip heights. Active in sports, good strength, no back pain or stiffness.

Objective. Spine straight without obvious deformities when erect, but mild right curvature of thoracic spine with forward flexion. No rib hump. Right shoulder and iliac crest slightly higher than left. Muscles and extremities symmetric; muscle strength appropriate and equal bilaterally; active range of motion without pain, locking, clicking, or limitation in all joints.

18

MERLIN mosby.com/MERLIN/Seidel

Neurologic System

EQUIPMENT

- Familiar objects (coins, keys, paper clip)
- Vials of aromatic substances (coffee, orange, peppermint, banana)
- Sterile needles
- Cotton wisp
- Tongue blades (one intact and one broken with point and rounded edges)
- List of tastes
- Vials of solutions (glucose, salt, lemon or vinegar, quinine) with applicators
- Cup of water
- Test tubes of hot and cold water
- Tuning forks
- Reflex hammer
- 5.07 monofilament

EXAMINATION

Evaluate the neurologic system as the rest of the body is examined. When history and examination findings have not revealed a potential neurologic problem, perform a neurologic screening examination as shown in box on p. 226, rather than a full neurologic examination. See Chapter 17, Musculoskeletal System, for evaluation of muscle tone and strength.

Cranial Nerves I-XII

Table on pp. 228-229 summarizes the cranial nerve (CN) examination. When a sensory or motor loss is suspected, be compulsive about determining the extent of the loss.

Neurologic Screening Examination

This shorter screening examination is commonly used for health visits when no known neurologic problem is apparent.

Cranial Nerves

Cranial nerves II through XII are routinely tested; however, taste and smell are not tested unless some aberration is found.

Proprioception and Cerebellar Function

One test is administered for each of the following: rapid rhythmic alternating movements, accuracy of movements, balance (Romberg test), gait and heel-toe walking.

Sensory Function

Superficial pain and touch at a distal point in each extremity are tested; vibration and position senses are assessed by testing the great toe.

Deep Tendon Reflexes

All deep tendon reflexes and the plantar reflex are tested, excluding the test for clonus.

TECHNIQUE	FINDINGS
Assess olfactory nerve (CN I)	
Ask patient to close eyes. Occlude one naris, hold vial (using least irritating aromatic substances first [e.g., orange or peppermint extract]) under nose, and ask patient to breathe deeply and identify odor. Allow patient to breathe comfortably, then occlude other naris and repeat with different odor. Continue, alternating two or three odors.	**EXPECTED:** Able to perceive and usually identify odor on each side. **UNEXPECTED:** Anosmia, loss of smell or inability to discriminate odors.
Assess optic nerve (CN II)	
See tests for visual acuity and visual fields in Chapter 7, Eyes.	

TECHNIQUE	FINDINGS

Assess oculomotor, trochlear, abducens nerves (CN III, CN IV, CN VI)

See tests for six cardinal points of gaze, pupil size, shape, response to light and accommodation, and opening of upper eyelids in Chapter 7, Eyes.

EXPECTED: Equal pupil size, equal and consensual response to light and accommodation, symmetric eye movements in all six cardinal points of gaze.

UNEXPECTED: Absence of lateral gaze. Absence of any expected findings, ptosis.

Assess trigeminal nerve (CN V)

■ *Facial muscle tone*
Ask patient to clench teeth tightly as you palpate muscles over jaw.

EXPECTED: Symmetric tone.
UNEXPECTED: Muscle atrophy, deviation of jaw to one side, or fasciculations.

■ *Sensation*
Ask patient to close eyes and report if sensation to touch is present or is sharp or dull as you touch each side of face at scalp, cheek, and chin areas, alternately using sharp and rounded edges of tongue blades or paper clip in an unpredictable pattern. Ask patient to report when the stimulus is felt as you stroke same six areas with cotton wisp or brush. Finally, test sensation over buccal mucosa with wooden applicator.

EXPECTED: Symmetric discrimination of sensations in each location to all stimuli.
UNEXPECTED: Impaired sensation. If impaired, use test tubes of hot and cold water to evaluate temperature sensation.

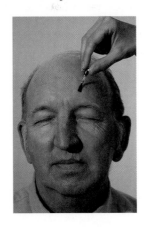

Procedures for Cranial Nerve Examination

Cranial Nerve (CN)	Procedure
CN I (olfactory)	Test ability to identify familiar aromatic odors, one naris at a time with eyes closed.
CN II (optic)	Test vision with Snellen chart and Rosenbaum near-vision chart.
	Perform ophthalmoscopic examination of fundi.
	Test visual fields by confrontation and extinction of vision.
CN III, CN IV, CN VI (oculomotor, trochlear, abducens)	Test extraocular movement.
	Inspect eyelids for drooping.
	Inspect pupil size for equality and direct and consensual response to light and accommodation.
CN V (trigeminal)	Inspect face for muscle atrophy and tremors.
	Palpate jaw muscles for tone and strength when patient clenches teeth.
	Test superficial pain and touch sensation in each branch.
	(Test temperature sensation if there are unexpected findings to pain or touch.)
	Test corneal reflex.
CN VII (facial)	Inspect symmetry of facial features with various expressions (e.g., smile, frown, puffed cheeks, wrinkled forehead).
	Test ability to identify sweet and salty tastes on each side of tongue.

CN VIII (acoustic)	Test sense of hearing with whisper screening tests or by audiometry.
	Compare bone and air conduction of sound.
	Test for lateralization of sound.
CN IX (glossopharyngeal)	Test ability to identify sour and bitter tastes.
	Test gag reflex and ability to swallow.
CN X (vagus)	Inspect palate and uvula for symmetry with speech sounds and gag reflex.
	Observe for swallowing difficulty.
	Evaluate quality of guttural speech sounds (presence of nasal or hoarse quality to voice).
CN XI (spinal accessory)	Test trapezius muscle strength (shrug shoulders against resistance).
	Test sternocleidomastoid muscle strength (turn head to each side against resistance).
CN XII (hypoglossal)	Inspect tongue in mouth and while protruded for symmetry, tremors, atrophy.
	Inspect tongue movement toward nose and chin.
	Test tongue strength with index finger when tongue is pressed against cheek.
	Evaluate quality of lingual speech sounds (*l, t, d, n*).

Modified from Rudy, 1984.

TECHNIQUE   FINDINGS

■ *Corneal reflex*
See test for corneal sensitivity
in Chapter 7, Eyes.

Assess facial nerve (CN VII)

■ *Expressions*
Ask patient to make following facial expressions:

- Raise eyebrows and wrinkle
  forehead
- Smile
- Frown
- Puff out cheeks
- Purse lips and blow out
- Show teeth
- Squeeze eyes shut against
  resistance

EXPECTED: Facial symmetry.
UNEXPECTED: Tics, unusual
facial movements, or asymmetry of expression (flattened na-
solabial fold, lower eyelid sag-
ging, side of mouth drooping).

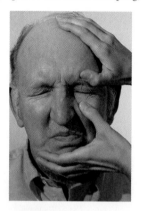

■ *Speech*

UNEXPECTED: Difficulties
with enunciating *b, m,* and *p*
(labial sounds).

■ *Taste (CN VII and CN IX)*
Hold card listing tastes in patient's view. Ask patient to extend tongue. Apply one of
four solutions to lateral side
of tongue in appropriate
taste-bud region. Ask patient
to point to taste perceived.

EXPECTED: Able to identify
sweet, salt, sour, bitter taste bilaterally when placed in appropriate taste-bud region.

TECHNIQUE   FINDINGS

Offer patient a sip of water, and repeat with different solution and applicator, testing each side of tongue with each solution.

Assess acoustic nerve (CN VIII)

- *Hearing*
  See screening tests in Chapter 8, Ears, Nose, and Throat.
- *Balance*
  See Romberg test, p. 234.

Assess glossopharyngeal nerve (CN IX)

- *Taste*
  See CN VII.
- *Gag reflex (nasopharyngeal sensation)*
  See CN X.

Assess vagus nerve (CN X)

- *Gag reflex (nasopharyngeal sensation) (CN IX and CN X)*
  Tell patient you will be testing gag reflex. Touch posterior wall of pharynx with applicator while observing palate, pharyngeal muscles, uvula.

  EXPECTED: Upward movement of palate and contraction of pharyngeal muscles, with uvula in midline.
  UNEXPECTED: Drooping or absence of arch on either side of soft palate; uvula deviates from midline.

- *Motor function*
  Ask patient to say "ah" while observing movement of soft palate and uvula.

  UNEXPECTED: Failure of soft palate to rise or deviation of uvula from midline.

- *Swallowing (CN IX and CN X)*
  Ask patient to swallow water.

  EXPECTED: Water easily swallowed.
  UNEXPECTED: Retrograde passage of water through nose.

TECHNIQUE	FINDINGS
■ Speech	**UNEXPECTED:** Hoarseness, nasal quality, or difficulty with guttural sounds.

Assess spinal accessory nerve (CN XI)

See Chapter 6, Head and Neck, and Chapter 17, Musculoskeletal System, for evaluations of size, shape, strength of trapezius and sternocleidomastoid muscles.

Assess hypoglossal nerve (CN XII)

■ *Tongue resting and protruded* Inspect while at rest on floor of mouth and while protruded.

EXPECTED: Tongue midline, symmetric size.
UNEXPECTED: Fasciculations, asymmetry, atrophy, or deviation from midline.

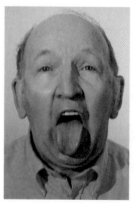

■ *Tongue movement* Ask patient to move tongue in and out, side to side, curled up toward nose, curled down toward chin.

EXPECTED: Able to perform most tongue movements.

■ *Tongue strength* Ask patient to push tongue against cheek while you apply resistance with index finger.

EXPECTED: Steady, firm pressure.

TECHNIQUE	FINDINGS

- *Speech*

UNEXPECTED: Problems with *l, t, d,* or *n* (lingual sounds).

Proprioception and Cerebellar Function

Evaluate coordination and fine motor skills

Have patient sit.

- *Rapid, rhythmic, alternating movements*
  Ask patient to pat knees with both hands, alternately patting with palms then backs of the hands. Alternatively, ask the patient to touch the thumb to each finger of the same hand sequentially from index finger to little finger and back, one hand at a time.

  EXPECTED: Smooth execution, maintaining rhythm with increasing speed.
  UNEXPECTED: Stiff, slowed, nonrhythmic, or jerky clonic movements.

- *Accuracy of movement: Finger-to-finger test*
  Position your index finger 40 to 50 cm from patient. Ask patient to alternately touch his or her nose and your index finger with the index finger of one hand, as shown below. Change location of your index finger several times. Repeat with patient's other hand.

  EXPECTED: Movements rapid, smooth, accurate.
  UNEXPECTED: Consistent past pointing (missing examiner's index finger).

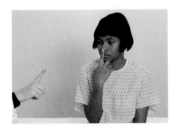
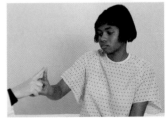

TECHNIQUE	FINDINGS

- *Accuracy of movement: Finger-to-nose test*
  Ask patient to close both eyes and touch his or her nose with index finger of each hand while alternating hands and gradually increasing speed.

  EXPECTED: Movements rapid, smooth, accurate, even with increasing speed.

- *Accuracy of movement: Heel-to-shin test* (can be performed sitting, standing, or supine)
  Ask patient to run heel of one foot along shin from knee to ankle of opposite leg. Repeat with other heel.

  EXPECTED: Able to move heel up and down shin in straight line.
  UNEXPECTED: Irregular deviations to side.

Evaluate balance

- *Balance: Romberg test*
  Ask patient to stand with feet together and arms at sides, with eyes first open, then closed. **Stand close by in case patient starts to fall.**

  EXPECTED: Slight swaying movement, no danger of falling.
  UNEXPECTED: Staggering, losing balance, or swaying to the extent of falling.

- *Balance: Recovery*
  After explaining test to patient, ask patient to spread feet slightly, then push shoulders to throw patient off balance. **Be prepared to catch patient.**

  EXPECTED: Quick recovery of balance.
  UNEXPECTED: Must catch patient to prevent a fall.

- *Balance: Standing and hopping*
  Have patient stand in place on one foot, then the other, with eyes open. Then have patient hop on each foot.

  EXPECTED: Able to stand and hop 5 seconds on each foot without losing balance.
  UNEXPECTED: Instability, need to continually touch floor with opposite foot, or tendency to fall.

TECHNIQUE	FINDINGS

- *Gait: Walking*
  Ask patient to walk without shoes around examining room or down hallway, with eyes first open, then closed.

EXPECTED: Smooth, regular gait rhythm and symmetric stride length; upright trunk posture swaying with gait phase; and arm swing smooth and symmetric.
UNEXPECTED: Shuffling, widely placed feet, toe walking, foot flop, leg lag, scissoring, loss of arm swing, staggering, lurching, or waddling motion.

- *Gait: Heel-toe walking*
  Ask patient to walk a straight line, first forward and then backward, with eyes open and arms at side. Ask patient to touch toe of one foot with heel of other.

EXPECTED: Consistent contact between toe and heel with slight swaying.
UNEXPECTED: Extension of arms for balance, instability, tendency to fall, or lateral staggering and reeling.

Sensory Function
Test primary sensory functions

Ask patient to close eyes for all tests. Use minimal stimulation initially, then increase gradually until patient becomes aware. Test contralateral areas, asking patient to compare perceived sensations side to side.

EXPECTED: For all tests, minimal differences side to side, correct interpretation of sensations, discrimination of side of body tested, location of sensation (e.g., proximal or distal to previous stimulus).
UNEXPECTED: For all tests, map boundaries of any impairment by distribution of major peripheral nerves or dermatomes (see figures on pp. 236-237).

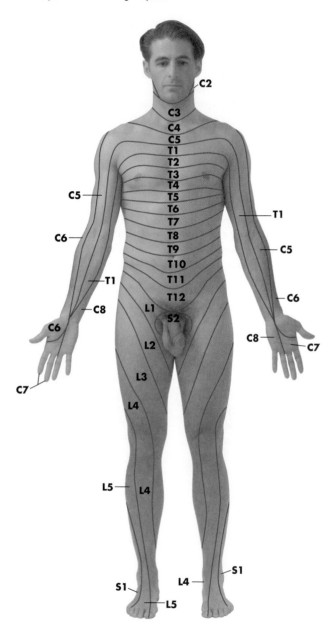

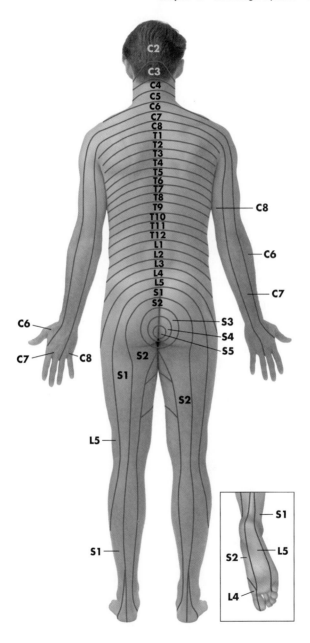

TECHNIQUE   FINDINGS

■ *Superficial touch*
Lightly touch skin with cotton wisp or your fingertips,
as shown at right. Ask patient
to point to area touched or
acknowledge when sensation
is felt.

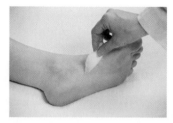

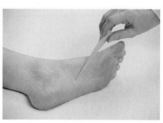

■ *Superficial pain*
Alternating sharp and
smooth edge of broken
tongue blade or point and
hub of sterile needle, touch
skin in unpredictable pattern.
Ask patient to identify sensation (sharp or dull) and
where it is felt.

■ *Temperature and deep pressure*
Perform test only if superficial pain sensation is not intact.
Temperature: Alternately roll
test tubes of hot and cold water against skin in an unpredictable pattern. Ask patient
to indicate hot or cold and
where it is felt.
Deep pressure: Squeeze   **EXPECTED:** Discomfort with
trapezius, calf, or biceps   deep pressure.
muscle.

TECHNIQUE	FINDINGS

■ *Protective sensation*
Perform test only if patient has diabetes mellitus or peripheral neuropathy. Apply 5.07 monofilament in a random pattern to several sites on plantar surface of foot and once on dorsal surface until filament bends. Avoid calloused areas and broken skin.

EXPECTED: Sensation felt at all sites touched.
UNEXPECTED: Loss of sensation at any site.

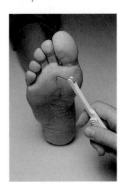

■ *Vibration*
Place stem of vibrating tuning fork against several bony prominences (e.g., toes, ankle, shin, finger joints, wrist, elbow, shoulder, sternum), beginning distally. Ask patient when and where sensation is felt and what it feels like. Dampen tines occasionally to see whether patient notices difference.

EXPECTED: Buzzing or tingling sensation.
UNEXPECTED: Does not distinguish vibration from touch of tuning fork.

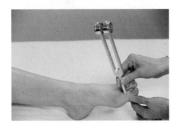

TECHNIQUE

FINDINGS

■ *Position of joints*
  Hold joint to be tested (great toe or finger) by lateral aspects in neutral position, then raise or lower digit, as shown, and ask patient which way it was moved. Return to neutral before moving in another direction. Repeat so both feet and both hands are tested.

EXPECTED: Patient correctly identifies position of joint.

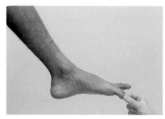

Test cortical sensory functions

Ask patient to close eyes for all tests.

■ *Stereognosis*
  Hand patient familiar objects (e.g., key, coin), and ask patient to identify.

UNEXPECTED: Inability to recognize objects (tactile agnosia).

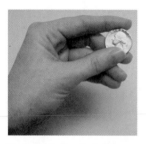

■ *Two-point discrimination*
  Using two sterile needles, alternately touch patient's skin with one or both points simultaneously at various locations. Find distance at which patient can no longer distinguish two points.

EXPECTED: See table on p. 241.

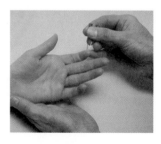

Minimal Distances of Discriminating Two Points

Body Part	Minimal Distance (mm)
Tongue	1
Fingertips	2-8
Toes	3-8
Palms of hands	8-12
Chest and forearms	40
Back	40-70
Upper arms and thighs	75

From Barkauskas et al, 2001.

TECHNIQUE

FINDINGS

- *Extinction phenomenon*
  Simultaneously touch cheek, hand, or other area on each side of body with sterile needles. Ask patient the number of stimuli and locations.

EXPECTED: Location of both sensations identified.

- *Graphesthesia*
  With blunt pen or applicator stick, draw letter or number on palm of patient's hand, and ask patient to identify it. Repeat with different figure on other hand.

EXPECTED: Letter or number readily recognized.

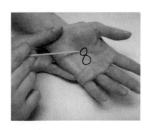

- *Point location*
  Touch area on patient's skin and withdraw stimulus. Ask patient to point to area touched.

EXPECTED: Able to locate stimulus.

TECHNIQUE   FINDINGS

Reflexes

Test superficial reflexes

Have patient supine.

■ *Abdominal*
Stroke each quadrant of abdomen with end of reflex
hammer or with tongue
blade edge.

EXPECTED: Slight, bilaterally
equal movement of umbilicus
toward each area of stimulation.

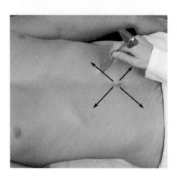

■ *Cremasteric (male patients)*
Stroke inner thigh, proximal
to distal.

EXPECTED: Testicle and scrotum rise on stroked side.

■ *Plantar reflex*
Using pointed object, stroke
lateral side of foot from heel
to ball, then curve across ball
to medial side.

EXPECTED: Plantar flexion of
all toes.
UNEXPECTED: Fanning of toes
or dorsiflexion of great toe with
or without fanning of other toes
(Babinski sign).

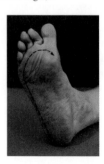

TECHNIQUE	FINDINGS

Test deep tendon reflexes

Patient relaxed and either sitting or lying for most procedures. Test each reflex, comparing responses on corresponding sides. Score deep tendon reflexes on scale shown in table on p. 244.

EXPECTED: Symmetric visible or palpable responses.
UNEXPECTED: Absent or diminished responses (0 or 1+), or hyperactive reflexes (3+ or 4+).

■ *Biceps*
Flex arm up 45 degrees at elbow, then palpate biceps tendon in antecubital fossa. Place thumb over tendon and fingers under elbow. Strike your thumb with reflex hammer.

EXPECTED: Visible or palpable flexion of elbow, contraction of biceps muscle.

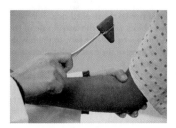

■ *Brachioradial*
Flex patient's arm up to 45 degrees while resting patient's forearm on your arm, with hand slightly pronated. Strike brachioradial tendon.

EXPECTED: Pronation of forearm and flexion of elbow.

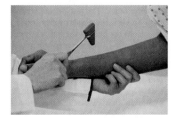

Scoring Deep Tendon Reflexes

Grade	Deep Tendon Reflex Response
0	No response
1+	Sluggish or diminished
2+	Active or expected response
3+	More brisk than expected, slightly hyperactive
4+	Brisk, hyperactive, with intermittent or transient clonus

TECHNIQUE

FINDINGS

- *Triceps*
  Flex patient's arm at elbow up to 90 degrees, and rest patient's hand against side of body. Palpate triceps tendon and strike directly with reflex hammer, just above elbow.

EXPECTED: Visible or palpable extension of elbow, contraction of triceps muscle.

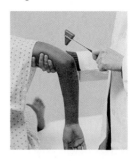

- *Patellar*
  Flex patient's knee up to 90 degrees, allowing lower leg to hang loosely. Support upper leg so it does not rest against edge of examining table, then strike patellar tendon just below patella.

EXPECTED: Extension of lower leg, contraction of quadriceps muscle.

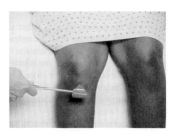

TECHNIQUE	FINDINGS

- *Achilles*
  Ask patient to sit. Then flex patient's knee and dorsiflex ankle up to 90 degrees, holding heel of foot. Strike Achilles tendon at level of ankle malleoli.

EXPECTED: Plantar flexion, contraction of gastrocnemius muscle.

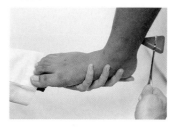

- *Clonus*
  Support patient's knee in partially flexed position and briskly dorsiflex foot with other hand, maintaining foot in flexion.

UNEXPECTED: Sustained clonus, rhythmic oscillating movements between dorsiflexion and plantar flexion palpated.

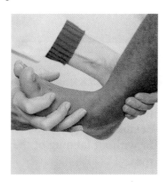

AIDS TO DIFFERENTIAL DIAGNOSIS

ABNORMALITY	DESCRIPTION
Generalized seizure disorder	Episodic, sudden, involuntary contractions of a group of muscles resulting from excessive discharge of cerebral neurons.

ABNORMALITY	DESCRIPTION
	Disturbances in conscious behavior, sensation, autonomic functioning, urinary and fecal incontinence may accompany seizures.
Meningitis	Inflammatory process of meninges. Fever, chills, nuchal rigidity, headache, seizures, vomiting, followed by alterations in level of consciousness. *Can be life threatening.*
Encephalitis	Inflammation of brain and spinal cord that often begins as a mild, febrile viral illness, often followed by a quiescent stage. Headache, drowsiness, confusion leading to stupor and coma. Possible motor function impairment with severe paralysis or ataxia.
Lesions (intracranial)	Headaches, vomiting, change in cognition, motor dysfunction, seizures, personality changes.
Cerebrovascular accident (brain attack or stroke)	Sudden, focal neurologic deficit resulting from impaired circulation of brain. Signs of headache, progressive changes in level of consciousness, vital sign and pupil changes, impaired communication.

ABNORMALITY	DESCRIPTION
Parkinson disease	Initial symptoms: Tremors at rest and with fatigue that disappear with intended movement and sleep. Progression tremor of head; slowing of voluntary movement; bilateral pill-rolling of fingers; delays in execution of movement; masked facial expression; poor blink rate; short, shuffling steps; slowed, slurred, monotonous speech; and possible behavioral changes and dementia.
Peripheral neuropathy	Decreased or loss of pain, vibratory, temperature sensation; absent reflexes and muscle wasting in affected extremity sometimes occurs.
Cerebral palsy	Alterations in muscle tone, posture, motor performance, reflexes, sensory impairment.

Clinical Signs of Motor Neuron Lesions

Upper Motor Neuron	Lower Motor Neuron
Muscle spasticity, possible contractures	Muscle flaccidity
Little or no muscle atrophy but decreased strength	Loss of muscle tone and strength; muscle atrophy
Hyperactive deep tendon and abdominal reflexes; absent plantar reflex	Weak or absent deep tendon, plantar, abdominal reflexes
No fasciculations	Fasciculations
Damage above level of brainstem will affect opposite side of body	Changes in muscles supplied by that nerve, usually a muscle on same side as the lesion
Paralysis of lower part of face, if involved	Bell palsy, if face involved; coordination unimpaired

PEDIATRIC VARIATIONS
EXAMINATION

Neurologic findings in infant and child change as child matures. For a complete description of anticipated maturational findings see Chapter 21.

TECHNIQUE	FINDINGS

Indirectly evaluate cranial nerves in newborns and infants

- *Optical blink reflex (CN II, CN III, CN IV, CN VI)*
  Shine a light at infant's open eyes. Observe quick closure of eyes and dorsal flexion of head.

  EXPECTED: Gazes intensely at close object or face. Focuses on and tracks an object with both eyes.
  UNEXPECTED: No response may indicate poor light perception.

- *Rooting reflex (CN V)*
  Touch one corner of infant's mouth.

  EXPECTED: Infant should open mouth and turn head in direction of stimulation. If infant has been fed recently, minimal or no response is expected.

- *Sucking reflex (CN V)*
  Place your finger in infant's mouth, feeling sucking action. Note pressure, strength, pattern of sucking.

  EXPECTED: Tongue should push up against your finger with good strength.

- *Infant's facial expression (CN VII)*
  Observe and note infant's ability to wrinkle forehead when crying and symmetry of smile.

  EXPECTED: Facial symmetry with all expressions.

- *Acoustic blink reflex (CN VIII)*
  Loudly clap your hands about 30 cm from infant's head; avoid producing an air current.

  EXPECTED: Blink in response to sound. Infant will habituate to repeated testing. Freezes position with high-pitched sound.

TECHNIQUE	FINDINGS
	UNEXPECTED: No response after 2 to 3 days of age may indicate hearing problems.
■ *Doll's eye maneuver (CN VIII)* Hold infant under axilla in upright position, head held steady, facing you. Rotate infant first in one direction and then in other.	**EXPECTED:** Infant's eyes should turn in direction of rotation and then opposite direction when rotation stops. **UNEXPECTED:** If eyes do not move in expected direction, suspect vestibular problem or eye muscle paralysis.
■ *Swallowing and gag reflex (CN IX and CN X)* ■ *Sucking and swallowing (CN XII)* Pinch infant's nose.	**EXPECTED:** Coordinated sucking and swallowing ability. Mouth will open, and tip of tongue will rise in midline position.

Evaluate primitive reflexes in infant

■ *Palmar grasp (present at birth)* Making sure infant's head is in midline, touch palm of infant's hand from ulnar side (opposite thumb).	**EXPECTED:** Strong grasp of your finger. Sucking facilitates grasp. Grasp should be strongest between 1 and 2 months of age and disappear by 3 months.
■ *Plantar grasp (present at birth)* Touch plantar surface of infant's feet at the base of toes.	**EXPECTED:** Toes should curl downward. Reflex should be strong up to 8 months of age.

TECHNIQUE	FINDINGS

- *Moro reflex (present at birth)*
  With infant supported in semisitting position, allow head and trunk to drop back to a 30-degree angle.

  EXPECTED: Symmetric abduction and extension of arms. Fingers fan out, and thumb and index finger form a C. Arms then adduct in an embracing motion followed by relaxed flexion. Reflex diminishes in strength by 3 to 4 months and disappears by 6 months.

- *Placing (4 days of age)*
  Hold infant upright under arms next to a table or chair. Touch dorsal side of foot to table or chair edge.

  EXPECTED: Flexion of hips and knees and lifting of foot as if stepping up on table. Age of disappearance varies.

- *Stepping (between birth and 8 weeks)*
  Hold infant upright under arms and allow soles of feet to touch surface of table.

  EXPECTED: Alternate flexion and extension of legs, simulating walking. Disappears before voluntary walking.

- *Asymmetric tonic neck or "fencing" (by 2 to 3 months)*
  With infant lying supine and relaxed or sleeping, turn infant's head to one side so jaw is over shoulder.

  EXPECTED: Extension of arm and leg on side to which head is turned and flexion of opposite arm and leg.

  Turn infant's head to other side.

  EXPECTED: Reversal of extremities' posture. Reflex diminishes at 3 to 4 months of age and disappears by 6 months.

  UNEXPECTED: Be concerned if infant never exhibits reflex or seems locked in fencing position.

Evaluate neurologic soft signs in children

Age (in years) at which finding becomes unexpected noted in parentheses.

- *Walking, running gait*

  UNEXPECTED: Stiff-legged with foot-slapping quality, unusual posturing of arm (3).

TECHNIQUE	FINDINGS
■ *Heel walking*	**UNEXPECTED:** Difficulty remaining on heels for distance of 10 feet (7).
■ *Tiptoe walking*	**UNEXPECTED:** Difficulty remaining on toes for distance of 10 feet (7).
■ *Tandem gait*	**UNEXPECTED:** Difficulty walking heel-to-toe, unusual posturing of arms (7).
■ *One-foot standing*	**UNEXPECTED:** Unable to remain standing on one foot longer than 5 to 10 seconds (5).
■ *Hopping in place*	**UNEXPECTED:** Unable to rhythmically hop on each foot (6).
■ *Motor-stance*	**UNEXPECTED:** Difficulty maintaining stance (arms extended in front, feet together, eyes closed), drifting of arms, mild writhing movements of hands or fingers (3).
■ *Visual tracking*	**UNEXPECTED:** Difficulty following object with eyes when keeping head still; nystagmus (5).
■ *Rapid thumb-to-finger test*	**UNEXPECTED:** Rapid touching of thumb to fingers in sequence is uncoordinated; unable to suppress mirror movements in contralateral hand (8).
■ *Rapid alternating movements of hands*	**UNEXPECTED:** Irregular speed and rhythm with pronation and supination of hands patting knees (10).
■ *Finger-nose test*	**UNEXPECTED:** Unable to alternately touch examiner's finger and own nose consecutively (7).

TECHNIQUE	FINDINGS
■ *Right-left discrimination*	**UNEXPECTED:** Unable to identify right and left sides of own body (5).
■ *Two-point discrimination*	**UNEXPECTED:** Difficulty in localizing and discriminating when touched in one or two places (6).
■ *Graphesthesia*	**UNEXPECTED:** Unable to identify geometric shapes drawn in child's open hand (8).
■ *Stereognosis*	**UNEXPECTED:** Unable to identify common objects placed in own hand (5).

Modified from Smith and McNamara, 1984.

SAMPLE DOCUMENTATION

Subjective. A 48-year-old man presents for his annual physical examination. No complaints of poor balance, loss of sensation, unsteady gait. History of diabetes mellitus type 1 for 30 years, well controlled.
Objective. Cranial nerves I to XII grossly intact. Gait is coordinated and even. Romberg test negative. Rapid alternating movements coordinated and smooth. Superficial touch, pain, vibratory sensation are intact bilaterally. Deep tendon reflexes 2+ bilaterally in all extremities. Babinski (plantar) reflex produces expected plantar flexion of toes. No ankle clonus. Monofilament test reveals decreased sensation on plantar surfaces of both feet.

19

Head-to-Toe Examination: Adult

COMPONENTS OF THE EXAMINATION

Because there is no one correct way to order the parts of the physical examination, you are encouraged to consider the following suggested approach for a particular setting, patient condition, or patient disability.

General Inspection

Start examination when patient is within your view. As you first observe patient, take note of following:

Signs of distress or disease
Habitus
Manner of sitting
Degree of relaxation on face
Relationship with others in room
Degree of interest in what is happening in room

On greeting patient, assess following:

Alacrity with which you are met
Moistness of palm when you shake hands
Eyes—luster and expression of emotion
Skin color
Facial expression
Mobility:
    Use of assistive devices
    Gait
    Sitting, rising from chair
    Taking off coat
Dress and posture

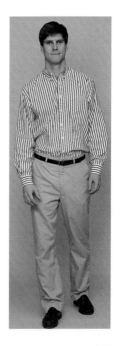

Speech pattern, disorders, foreign language
Difficulty hearing, assistive devices
Stature and build
Musculoskeletal deformities
Vision problems, assistive devices
Eye contact with you
Orientation, mental alertness
Nutritional state
Respiratory problems
Significant others accompanying patient

Patient Instructions

Empty bladder.
Remove as much clothing as is necessary.
Put on a gown.

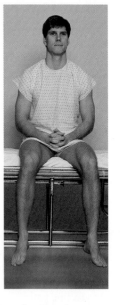

Measurements

Measure height.
Measure weight.
Assess distance vision—Snellen chart.
Document vital signs—temperature,
   pulse, respiration, blood pressure in
   both arms.

Patient Seated, Wearing Gown

Stand in front of patient seated on examining table.

Head and face

Inspect skin characteristics.
Inspect symmetry and external characteristics of eyes and ears.
Inspect configuration of skull.
Inspect and palpate scalp and hair for texture, distribution, quan-
   tity of hair.
Palpate facial bones.
Palpate temporomandibular joint while patient opens and closes
   mouth.
Palpate sinus regions; if tender, transilluminate.
Inspect ability to clench teeth, squeeze eyes tightly shut, wrinkle
   forehead, smile, stick out tongue, puff out cheeks (cranial
   nerve [CN] V, CN VII).
Test light sensation of forehead, cheeks, chin (CN V).

Eyes

External examination:
Inspect eyelids, eyelashes, palpebral folds.
Determine alignment of eyebrows.
Inspect sclerae, conjunctivae, irides.
Palpate lacrimal apparatus.
Near-vision screening—Rosenbaum chart (CN II).
Eye function:
Test pupillary response to light and accommodation.
Perform cover-uncover test and light reflex.
Test extraocular eye movements (CN III, CN IV, CN VI).
Assess visual fields (CN II).
Test corneal reflexes (CN V).
Ophthalmoscopic examination:
Test red reflex.
Inspect lens.
Inspect disc, cup margins, vessels, retinal surface, vitreous humor.

Ears

Inspect alignment and placement.
Inspect surface characteristics.
Palpate auricle.
Assess hearing with whisper test (CN VIII).
Perform otoscopic examination:
Inspect canals.
Inspect tympanic membranes for landmarks, deformities, inflammation.
Use a tuning fork to assess bone and air conduction.

Nose

Note structure, position of septum.
Determine patency of each nostril.
Inspect mucosa, septum, turbinates with nasal speculum.
Assess olfactory function when indicated: Test sense of smell (CN I).

Mouth and pharynx

Inspect lips, buccal mucosa, gums, hard and soft palates, floor of mouth for color and surface characteristics.
Inspect oropharynx: Note anteroposterior pillars, uvula, tonsils, posterior pharynx, mouth odor.

Inspect teeth for color, number, surface characteristics.

Inspect tongue for color, characteristics, symmetry, movement (CN XII).

Test gag reflex and "ah" reflex (CN IX, CN X).

Perform sense of taste test (CN VII, CN IX) when indicated.

Neck

Inspect for symmetry and smoothness of neck and thyroid.

Inspect for jugular venous distention.

Perform active and passive range of motion; test resistance against examiner's hand.

Test strength of shoulder shrug (CN XI).

Palpate carotid pulses. Be sure to palpate one side at a time.

Palpate tracheal position.

Palpate thyroid.

Palpate lymph nodes—preauricular and postauricular, occipital, tonsillar, submental, submandibular, superficial cervical chain, posterior cervical, deep cervical, supraclavicular.

Auscultate carotid arteries and thyroid.

Upper extremities

Observe and palpate hands, arms, shoulders.

    Skin and nail characteristics

    Muscle mass

    Muscular strength

    Musculoskeletal deformities

    Joint range of motion—fingers, wrists, elbows, shoulders

Assess pulses—radial, brachial.

Palpate epitrochlear nodes.

Patient Seated, Back Exposed

Stand behind patient seated on examining table.

Have males pull gown down to the waist so entire chest and back are exposed.

Have females expose back; keep breasts covered.

Back and posterior chest

Inspect skin and thoracic configuration.

Inspect symmetry of shoulders, musculoskeletal development.

Inspect and palpate scapulae and spine.

Palpate and percuss costovertebral angle.

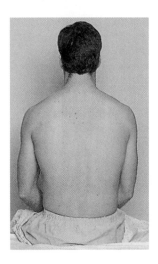

Lungs

Inspect respiration—excursion, depth, rhythm, pattern.

Palpate for expansion and tactile fremitus.

Palpate scapular and subscapular nodes.

Percuss posterior chest and lateral walls systematically for resonance.

Percuss for diaphragmatic excursion.

Auscultate systematically for breath sounds (egophony, bronchophony, whispered pectoriloquy): Note characteristics and adventitious sounds.

Patient Seated, Chest Exposed

Move around to front of patient.

Have females lower gown to expose anterior chest.

Anterior chest, lungs, heart

Inspect skin, musculoskeletal development, symmetry.

Inspect respirations—patient posture, respiratory effort.

Inspect for pulsations or heaving.

Palpate chest wall for stability, crepitation, tenderness.

Palpate precordium for thrills, heaves, pulsations.

Palpate left chest to locate apical impulse.

Palpate for tactile fremitus.

Palpate nodes—infraclavicular, axillary.

Percuss systematically for breath sounds.

Auscultate systematically for breath sounds.

Auscultate systematically for heart sounds—aortic area, pulmonic area, second pulmonic area, tricuspid area, mitral area.

Female breasts

Inspect in these positions—patient's arms extended over head, pushing hands on hips, hands pushed together in front of chest, patient leaning forward.

Palpate breasts in all four quadrants, tail of Spence, over areolae; if breasts are large, perform bimanual palpation.

Palpate nipple: Compress to observe for discharge.

Male breasts

Inspect breasts and nipples for symmetry, enlargement, surface characteristics.

Palpate breast tissue.

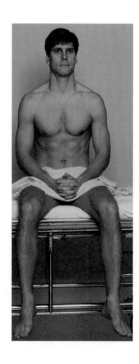

Patient Reclining 45 Degrees

Assist patient to a reclining position at a 45-degree angle.
Stand to side of patient that allows greatest comfort.
Inspect chest in recumbent position.
Inspect jugular venous pulsations; measure jugular venous pressure.

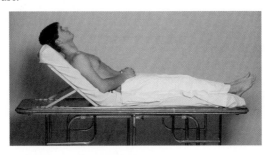

Patient Supine, Chest Exposed

Assist patient into supine position.
If patient cannot tolerate lying flat, maintain head elevation at
30-degree angle.
Uncover chest while keeping abdomen and lower extremities
draped.

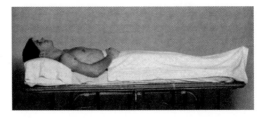

Female breasts

Inspect and palpate with patient in recumbent position.
Palpate systematically with patient's arm over her head and with
her arm at her side.

Heart

Palpate chest wall for thrills, heaves, pulsations.
Auscultate systematically; turn patient slightly to left side and repeat auscultation.

Patient Supine, Abdomen Exposed

Have patient remain supine.
Cover chest with patient's gown.
Arrange draping to expose abdomen from pubis to epigastrium.

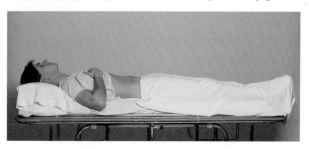

Abdomen

Inspect skin characteristics, contour, pulsations, movement.
Auscultate all quadrants for bowel sounds.
Auscultate aorta and renal, iliac, and femoral arteries for bruits or
   venous hums.
   Percuss all quadrants for tone.
   Percuss liver borders and estimate span.
Percuss left midaxillary line for splenic dullness.
Lightly palpate all quadrants.
Deeply palpate all quadrants.
   Palpate right costal margin for liver border.
   Palpate left costal margin for spleen.
   Palpate for right and left kidneys.
   Palpate midline for aortic pulsation.
Test abdominal reflexes.
Have patient raise head as you inspect abdominal muscles.

Inguinal area

Palpate for lymph nodes, pulses, hernias.

External genitalia, males

Inspect penis, urethral meatus, scrotum, pubic hair.
Palpate scrotal contents (you may want to have patient assume an
   alternate position, such as standing or sitting).

Patient Supine, Legs Exposed

Have patient remain supine.

Arrange drapes to cover abdomen and pubis and to expose lower
  extremities.

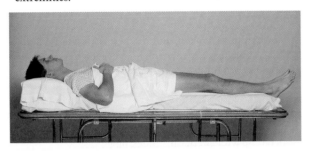

Feet and legs

Inspect for skin characteristics, hair distribution, muscle mass,
  musculoskeletal configuration.

Palpate for temperature, texture, edema, pulses (dorsalis pedis,
  posterior tibial, popliteal).

Test range of motion and strength of toes, feet, ankles, knees.

Hips

Palpate hips for stability.

Test range of motion and strength of hips.

Patient Sitting, Lap Draped

Assist patient to a sitting position.

Have patient wear gown with a drape across lap.

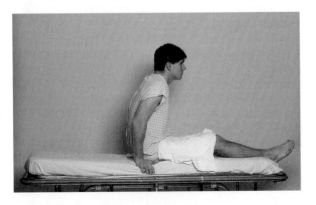

Musculoskeletal

Observe patient moving from lying to sitting position.
Note coordination, use of muscles, muscle strength, ease of movement.

Neurologic

Test sensory function—dull and sharp sensation of forehead, cheeks, chin, lower arms, hands, lower legs, feet.
Test vibratory sensation of wrists, ankles.
Test two-point discrimination of palms, thighs, back.
Test stereognosis, graphesthesia.
Test fine motor function, coordination, and position sense of upper extremities, asking patient to do following:
  Touch nose with alternating index fingers.
  Rapidly alternate touching fingers to thumb.
  Rapidly move index finger between own nose and examiner's finger.
Test fine motor function, coordination, and position sense of lower extremities, asking patient to do following:
  Run heel down tibia of opposite leg.
  Alternately and rapidly cross leg over opposite knee.
Test deep tendon reflexes and compare bilaterally—biceps, triceps, brachioradial, patellar, Achilles.
Test plantar reflex bilaterally.

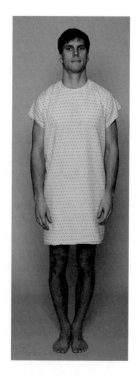

Patient Standing

Assist patient to standing position.
Stand next to patient.

Spine

Inspect and palpate spine as patient bends over at waist.
Test range of motion—hyperextension, lateral bending, rotation of upper trunk.

Neurologic

Observe gait.

Test proprioception and cerebellar function:

Perform Romberg test.

Ask patient to walk heel to toe.

Ask patient to stand on one foot, then the other, with eyes closed.

Ask patient to hop in place on one foot, then other.

Ask patient to do deep knee bends.

Abdominal/genital

Test for inguinal and femoral hernias.

Female Patient, Lithotomy Position

Assist female patient into lithotomy position, and drape appropriately.

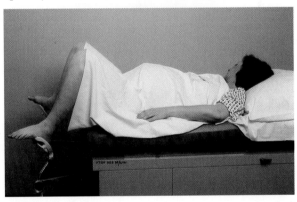

Sit at end of examining table.

External genitalia

Inspect pubic hair, labia, clitoris, urethral opening, vaginal opening, perineal and perianal area, anus.

Palpate labia and Bartholin glands; milk Skene glands.

Internal genitalia

Perform speculum examination:

Inspect vagina and cervix.

Collect Pap smear and other necessary specimens.

Perform bimanual palpation to assess for characteristics of vagina, cervix, uterus, adnexa.

Perform rectovaginal examination to assess rectovaginal septum, broad ligaments.

Perform rectal examination:

Assess anal sphincter tone and surface characteristics.

Obtain rectal culture if needed.

Note characteristics of stool when gloved finger is removed.

Male Patient, Bending Forward

Assist male patient in leaning over examining table or into knee-chest position. Stand behind patient.

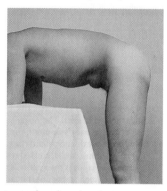

Inspect sacrococcygeal and perianal areas.

Perform rectal examination:

Palpate sphincter tone and surface characteristics.

Obtain rectal culture if needed.

Palpate prostate gland and seminal vesicles.

Note characteristics of stool when gloved finger is removed.

Examination Conclusion

Allow patient to dress in private.

Share findings and interpretations with patient.

Answer any of patient's additional questions.

Confirm that patient has a clear understanding of all aspects of the situation.

If patient is examined in a hospital bed:

Put everything back in order when finished.

Make sure patient is comfortably settled in an appropriate manner.

Put bed side rails up if clinical condition warrants it.

Make sure buttons and buzzers are within easy reach.

The Healthy Female Evaluation

Following are items to consider for inclusion as part of a routine well-woman visit. This is not intended as an all-inclusive list. Some items may vary depending on the woman's age, health status, and particular risk factors. Past medical history (PMH) and review of systems (ROS) may also be appropriate if indicated. Age and risk-status guidelines for preventive services are available from a variety of sources and authorities.*

HISTORY
History of Present Illness (HPI)

Age

Last normal menstrual period (LNMP)

Menopause—age achieved, symptoms

Obstetric history—number of pregnancies, term pregnancies, preterm pregnancies, abortions/miscarriages, living children (GPTAL)

Contraceptive measures and history

Sexual history

Unusual vaginal bleeding or discharge

---

*U.S. Preventive Services Task Force: *Guide to clinical preventive services,* ed 2, Washington, DC, 1996, The Task Force; U.S. Department of Health and Human Services: *Clinician's handbook of preventive services,* Washington, DC, 1994, The Department.

Authorities that produce prevention guidelines include Academy of Family Physicians, American Cancer Society, American College of Obstetricians and Gynecologists, American College of Physicians, American Geriatrics Society, Canadian Task Force on the Periodic Health Examination, National Cancer Institute, and U.S. Preventive Services Task Force.

Abdominal or pelvic pain
Urinary symptoms

Risk Assessment

Cardiovascular—smoking, hypertension, diet, body mass index (BMI), exercise, family history
Cancer—personal/family history of breast, ovarian, or colon cancer; history of sun exposure
Infection—sexually transmitted disease (STD) exposure; tuberculosis exposure; hepatitis vaccine or exposure; last tetanus immunization
Metabolic—calcium supplement, family history of osteoporosis; exercise; personal/family history of diabetes mellitus
Injury—alcohol, seat belts, guns, family violence
Depression—vegetative symptoms (eating, sleeping, concentration, energy, social interaction)

Health Habits

Breast self-examination
Pap smear—how often, date of last Pap smear; results, ever an abnormal result
Mammogram—date, result of last mammogram
Diet—fat, cholesterol, calcium
Exercise
Smoking
Alcohol/drugs

PHYSICAL EXAMINATION

Vital signs
Height and weight; BMI
Skin—lesions, moles
Lungs
Cardiovascular and peripheral vascular
Breasts—contour, masses, nipple discharge
Lymph—regional lymphadenopathy (infraclavicular and supraclavicular, axillary)
Abdomen—bowel sounds, masses, organ enlargement, hernias
Pelvic—lesions, discharge; Bartholin glands, urethra, Skene glands; vagina, cervix, adnexa, uterus
Rectal—hemorrhoids, masses, lesions

SCREENING TESTS

Pap smear—frequency depends on age, sexual status, PMH, Pap smear history

STD testing—depending on exposure status

Mammogram—frequency depends on age, personal and family history, past results

Fecal occult blood test or flexible sigmoidoscopy or colonoscopy—depending on age, personal and family history

Cholesterol/lipid profile—depending on age, personal and family history

Clinical and Reference Notes

21

Age-Specific Examination: Infants, Children, and Adolescents

EXAMINATION GUIDELINES

The approach to a pediatric physical examination must, of course, be age appropriate. Not every observation must be made in every child at every examination. What you do depends on the individual circumstance and on your clinical judgment. Each step must be considered in relation to the patient's age, physical condition, and emotional state. The order of the examination can be modified according to need; it should not be stereotypical. Care should be given to ensure the safety of the child on the examining table. During the pre–elementary school years (and sometimes later), an adult's lap is often a better site for much and often all of the examination.

Your notes should include a description of child's behavior during interactions with parent (or surrogate) and with you.

Take child's temperature, weight, length or height. Take blood pressure and record extremity or extremities used, size of cuff, and method used.

Note percentiles for all measurements.

Depending on clinical requirements, consider including arm span, upper segment measurement (crown to top of symphysis), lower segment measurement (symphysis to soles of feet), upper/lower segment ratio, head and chest circumference.

Offer toys or paper and pencil to entertain child (if age appropriate), to develop rapport, and to evaluate development, motor and neurologic status.

Use a developmental screening test such as Denver II to evaluate language, motor coordination, social skills.

Evaluate mental status as child interacts with you and parent.
Take advantage of opportunities child presents during examination to make your observations.

Child Playing

While child plays on the floor, evaluate musculoskeletal and neurologic systems while developing a rapport with child.

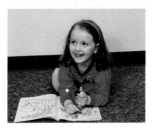

Observe child's spontaneous activities.
Ask child to demonstrate skills such as throwing a ball, building block towers, drawing geometric figures, coloring.
Evaluate gait, jumping, hopping, range of motion.
Muscle strength: Observe child climbing on parent's lap, stooping, and recovering.

Child on Parent's Lap

Perform examination on parent's lap to enhance child's participation.
Begin with child sitting and undressed except for diaper or underpants.

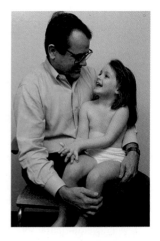

Upper extremities

Inspect arms for movement, size, shape; observe use of hands; inspect hands for number and configuration of fingers, palmar creases.
Palpate radial pulses.
Elicit biceps and triceps reflexes when child cooperates.

Take blood pressure at this point or later, depending on child's attitude.

Lower extremities

Child may stand for much or part of examination.
Inspect legs for movement, size, shape, alignment, lesions.
Inspect feet for alignment, longitudinal arch, number of toes.
Palpate femoral and dorsalis pedis pulses.
Elicit plantar reflex and, if child is cooperative, Achilles and patellar reflexes.

Head and neck

Inspect head.
Inspect shape, alignment with neck, hairline, position of auricles.
Palpate anterior fontanel for size; head for sutures, depressions; hair for texture.
Measure head circumference.
Inspect neck for webbing, voluntary movement.
Palpate neck: Position of trachea, thyroid, muscle tone, lymph nodes.

Chest, heart, lungs

Inspect chest for respiratory movement, size, shape, precordial movement, deformity, nipple and breast development.
Palpate anterior chest, locate point of maximal impulse, note tactile fremitus in talking or crying child.
Auscultate anterior, lateral, and posterior chest for breath sounds; count respirations.
Auscultate all cardiac listening areas for S_1 and S_2, splitting, murmurs; count apical pulse.

Child Relatively Supine, Still on Lap, Diaper Loosened

Inspect abdomen.
Auscultate for bowel sounds.
Palpate: Identify size of liver and any other palpable organs or masses.
Percuss.
Palpate femoral pulses; compare with radial pulses.
Palpate for lymph nodes.

Inspect external genitalia.

Males: Palpate scrotum for descent of testes and other masses.

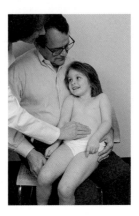

Child Standing

Inspect spinal alignment as child bends slowly forward to touch toes.

Observe posture from anterior, posterior, lateral views.

Observe gait.

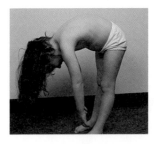

Child on Parent's Lap

Prepare child for examination

Only if absolutely necessary, restrain child for funduscopic, otoscopic, oral examinations.

Lessen fear of these examinations by permitting child to handle instruments, blow out light, or use them on a doll or on parent.

Attempt to gain child's cooperation, even if it takes more time; future visits will be more pleasant for both of you.

After finishing these preliminary maneuvers, perform the following:

Inspect eyes: Corneal light reflex, red reflex, extraocular movements, funduscopic examination.

Perform otoscopic examination. Note position and description of pinnae.

Inspect nasal mucosa.

Inspect mouth and pharynx. Note number of teeth, deciduous or permanent, and any special characteristics.

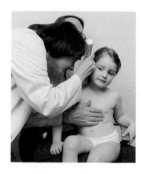

(NOTE: By the time child is of school age, it is usually possible to use an examination sequence very similar to that for adults.) See pp. 292-299 for examples of forms used to chart physical growth.

AGE-SPECIFIC ANTICIPATED OBSERVATIONS AND GUIDELINES*

Keep in mind that this is a suggested outline, always modified by human variation, and that all percentages are subject to gaussian distribution. History taking can be facilitated by referring to baby books, report cards, pictures, and other materials the family may have at home. Also, these suggestions assume a continuing relationship with the patient. Of course, you must begin with a full history and physical examination at whatever age you first see the patient.

---

*Adapted from clinic forms used in the Primary Care Continuity Clinic in the Children's Medical Center at The Johns Hopkins Hospital under the leadership of Drs. Janet Servint and Kevin Johnson and from the pediatric section, authored by Henry M. Seidel, of "Clinical History and Physical Examination," a booklet prepared for second-year medical students at The Johns Hopkins School of Medicine under the direction of Lawrence S. C. Griffith, MD.

2 Weeks of Age

History (particular attention)

Pertinent perinatal history
Social: Sleeping arrangements, housing
Stool pattern
Umbilicus: Healing, discharge, granulation
Diet: Feeding modality, schedule

Development: By this age

80% will lift and turn head when in prone position
40% will follow an object to midline visually
35% will vocalize, become quiet in response to a voice
45% will regard a face intently, diminishing activity for the moment

Physical examination (particular attention)

Establish growth curves (weight, height, head circumference).
Examine hips.
Test reflexes: Moro, root, grasp, step.

Anticipatory guidance (particular attention)

Sleep (emphasize supine position and avoidance of soft and fuzzy threats to safe breathing)
Feeding: Use of pacifier (need to suck)
Use of bulb syringe (nasal stuffiness)
Safety: Falling, crib sides, car seats
Skin care
Clothing
Illness: Temperature taking
Crying (holding the baby)

Plans and problems

What risks have revealed themselves as you got to know the family? What are apparent problems? Start a problem list and make appropriate dispositions.
Consider need for hemoglobin or hematocrit value.
Consider immunization needs and, throughout, attempt to follow American Academy of Pediatrics guidelines; on each visit, discuss benefits, risks, side effects of immunizations (always remember risks for the immunocompromised).

2 Months of Age

History (particular attention)

Expressions of parental concern
Child's apparent temperament
Sleep cycle
Feeding patterns, frequency
Stooling pattern, frequency, color, consistency, straining
Be certain there is no probability of immunocompromise in patient or relevant family members or other contacts (before starting immunizations)
Social issues:
  Father's involvement
  Living conditions
  Smoking, other concerning habits
  Any apparent high-risk concerns

Development: By this age

Gross motor:
  80% will lift head to 45 degrees in prone position
  45% will lift head to as much as 90 degrees in prone position
  25% will roll over stomach to back
Fine motor:
  99%+ will follow a moving object to midline
  85% will follow a moving object past midline
Language:
  Almost all will diminish activity at the sound of a voice
  35% will spontaneously vocalize
  Many will vocalize responsively
Psychosocial:
  Almost all will diminish activity when regarding a face
  Almost all will respond to a friendly, cooing face with a social smile
  50% may smile spontaneously or even laugh aloud

Physical examination (particular attention)

Growth curves (weight, height, head circumference)
Hearing
Vision
Hips

Anticipatory guidance

Feeding (delay or at least downplay solids; avoid citrus, wheat, mixed foods, eggs; minimize water)

When and if mother returns to work

Hiccups

Straining at stool

Visual and auditory stimulus (mobiles, mirrors, rattles, singing and talking to baby)

Sibling rivalry (if there are siblings)

Babysitters (checking references, ensuring immunization status, reliability)

Safety (rolling over, playpen, car seat, discourage walker, no smoking)

Sleep (reemphasize location and supine position)

Smoking and contribution to poor health

Plans and problems

Review immunizations, and implement as appropriate.

List problems (e.g., allergies, medications, any areas of concern), and make appropriate plans and, when necessary, referrals.

Consider need for hemoglobin or hematocrit value.

4 Months of Age

History (particular attention)

Parental concerns

Infant's sleep cycle and temperament

Feeding patterns, frequency, mother's feelings if she is breast-feeding

Stooling pattern, frequency, color, consistency, straining

Social issues:

Father's involvement

Amplification of early impressions of home's social structure

Smoking, other concerning habits

Any apparent high-risk concerns

Development: By this age

Gross motor:

80%, when prone, will lift chest up with arm support

80% will roll over from stomach to back

35% will have no head lag when pulled to sitting position, and many will then hold head steady when kept in that position

Fine motor:
   60% will reach for a dangling object
   Almost all will bring hands together
   Almost all will follow a face or object up to 180 degrees
Language:
   Almost all will laugh aloud
   20% will appear to initiate vocalization
Psychosocial:
   80% will smile spontaneously
   Many will regard their own hand for several seconds

Physical examination (particular attention)

Update growth curves (weight, height, head circumference).
Reassess hearing.
Reassess vision.

Anticipatory guidance

Introduction of solid food (cereal)
Stool changes with changes in diet
Drooling and teething
Thumb sucking, pacifiers, bottles at bedtime
Safety (aspiration, rolling over, holding baby with hot liquids,
   reemphasize earlier discussions [e.g., car seat])
Reemphasis on environmental stimulus
Further discussion of babysitters
Use of antipyretics (e.g., acetaminophen)

Plans and problems

Review immunizations and implement as appropriate.
Maintain problem list, making appropriate plans and, if neces-
   sary, referrals.
Consider need for hematocrit or hemoglobin value.

6 Months of Age

History (interim details)

Parental concerns
Sleep patterns
Diet
Stooling pattern
Further exploration of social issues
 If either parent has not attended these care visits regularly, en-
   courage his or her participation, and address relevant issues

Development: By this age

Gross motor:
90%, pulled to a sitting position, will have no head lag
60% will sit alone
75% will bear some weight on legs
Almost all will roll over

Fine motor:
More than half will pass a toy from hand to hand
60%, in a sitting position, will look for a toy
40%, in a sitting position, will take two cubes

Language:
60% will turn toward a voice
30% will initiate speech sounds (e.g., *mama, dada*) but not specifically

Psychosocial:
30% may cry and turn away from strangers
40% may put an object in mouth to explore it, may feed self
60%, holding an object, may resist an attempt to pull it away

Physical examination (particular attention)

Update growth curves.
Double-check hearing and vision.
Look for any new findings, and recheck the old.

Anticipatory guidance

Bedtime routines (discuss putting child to bed while she is awake; waking up at night)
Fear of strangers
Separation anxiety
Safety (begin discussions about what toddlers can get into, cabinets, hot water, electrical outlets, medications and other poisons; inform about local poison control center, syrup of ipecac)
Shoes, when and if to use them
Teething, oral hygiene
Offering a cup
Checking fluoride intake
Addition of solid foods

Plans and problems

Review immunizations and implement as appropriate.

Consider need for a serum lead level, hemoglobin or hematocrit value.

Maintain problem list, making appropriate plans and, if necessary, referrals.

9 Months of Age

History (interim details)

Parental concerns
Continued attention to sleep, diet, stooling patterns
Continuing attention to social issues

Development: By this age

Gross motor:
Almost 100% will sit alone
80% will stand alone
45% will cruise
Some will have begun competent crawling
Fine motor:
70% will have thumb-finger grasp
60% will bang two cubes together
Almost all will finger feed
Language:
75% will imitate speech sounds
75% will use *mama, dada* nonspecifically
Psychosocial:
Almost 100% will try to get to a toy that is out of reach
85% will play repetitive games (e.g., peek-a-boo)
45% will be shy with strangers and may cry

Physical examination (particular attention)

Update growth curves.
Constantly reassess earlier findings, and look for anything new.

Anticipatory guidance

Oral hygiene, for example, water without sugar in bottles (avoid tooth decay)
Sleep and desirability of routine (naps, separation anxiety and how to deal with it)
Reemphasis on babysitters, references and reliability
Safety, for example, stair gates and toddlers, falls, poisoning, burns, aspiration (never enough emphasis on safety, smoking, etc.)

Weaning, breast and/or bottle

Uses of discipline

Plans and problems

Review immunizations, and implement as appropriate.

Consider need for a serum lead level, hemoglobin, or hematocrit value.

Maintain problem list, making appropriate plans and, if necessary, referrals.

12 Months of Age

History (interim details)

Assess parental concerns.

Reassess social and system review.

Development: By this age

Gross motor:

85% will cruise

70% will stand alone briefly

50% will walk to some extent, and more will try it with hands held

Fine motor:

90% will bang two cubes together

70% will have a good pincer grasp

Language:

80% will use *mama* and *dada* specifically

30% will use as many as three additional words

Almost all will indulge in immature jargoning

Psychosocial:

Almost all will respond to parent's presence and voice

Almost all will wave bye-bye

85% will play pat-a-cake

50% will drink from a cup

About half, perhaps a bit more, will play ball with examiner

Physical examination (particular attention)

Update growth curves.

Continue reassessment.

Evaluate gait if walking has begun.

Anticipatory guidance

Reduced food intake in many (this is expected)
Weaning (especially at night)
Increased use of table food
Dental health, toothbrushing
Toilet training (expectations, attitudes)
Discipline (e.g., limit setting)
Safety (child-proofing house, street, lead paint, etc.)

Plans and problems

Review immunizations and implement as appropriate.
Consider need for a serum lead level, hemoglobin or hematocrit value, tuberculosis test.
Maintain problem list, making appropriate plans and, if necessary, referrals.

15 Months of Age

History (interim details)

Assess parental concerns.
Reassess social and system review.

Development: By this age

Gross motor:
   Almost all will walk well
   Almost all will stoop to recover an object
   35% will walk up steps with help
Fine motor:
   Almost all will drink from a cup
   Almost all will have a neat pincer grasp
   70% will scribble with crayon
   60% will make a tower with two cubes
Language:
   Almost all will use *mama* and *dada* specifically
   75% will use as many as three additional words
   30% will put two words together
Psychosocial:
   Many more than 50% will play ball with examiner
   50% will try to use a spoon
   45% will try to remove clothing

Physical examination (particular attention)

Update growth curves.
Continued reassessment.
Evaluate gait.

Anticipatory guidance

Negativism and independence
Dental health (visit to a dentist)
Toilet training
Weaning
Discipline (e.g., need for consistency)
Safety (all issues, repetitively)

Plans and problems

Review immunizations and implement as appropriate.
Consider need for a serum lead level, hemoglobin or hematocrit value, tuberculosis test.
Maintain problem list, making appropriate plans and, if necessary, referrals.

18 Months of Age

History (interim details)

Assess parental concerns.
Reassess social and system review.

Development: By this age

Gross motor:
    55% will have begun to walk up stairs without much help
    70% will have started to walk backwards
    More than that will have tried running with at least some success
    45% will have tried with some success to kick a ball forward, given the opportunity
Fine motor:
    80% will scribble if given a crayon
    80% will make a tower with two cubes
    About half of those will attempt with some success a tower of even as many as four cubes
Language:
    Almost all will have mature jargoning

85% will have at least three words in addition to *mama* and *dada*

Many of those will put two words together

More than half will respond to a one-step command (e.g., when asked to point to a body part)

Psychosocial:

Well over half will assist with taking off their clothes

75% will use a spoon successfully, albeit with some spillage

Physical examination (particular attention)

Update growth curves.

Continue reassessment; search for new findings.

Continue to evaluate gait.

Anticipatory guidance

Sleep (naps, nightmares)

Diet (mealtime battles)

Dental health (toothbrushing, dentist)

Toilet training

Discipline (methods and, again, consistency)

Safety (never enough discussion [e.g., seat belt, street and car, childproofing home])

Self-comforting (masturbation, thumb sucking, favorite blankets and toys)

Child care settings if one is necessary

Plans and problems

Review immunizations and implement as appropriate.

Consider need for serum lead level, hemoglobin or hematocrit value, tuberculosis test.

Maintain problem list, making appropriate plans and, if necessary, referrals.

2 Years of Age

History (interim details)

Assess parental concerns.

Reassess social and system review.

Development: By this age

Gross motor:

All should run well

All should walk up steps of reasonable height without holding on

90% will kick a ball forward

80% will throw a ball overhand

60% will do a little jump

40% may balance on one foot for 1 to 2 seconds

Fine motor:

Almost all should scribble with a pencil

90% will make a tower of four cubes

70% will copy a vertical line

Language:

All should point to and name parts of body

85% will readily combine two different words

80% will understand *on* and *under*

75% will name a picture

Psychosocial:

85% will give a toy to mother or other significant person

60% will put on some clothing alone and, often, also remove a garment

50% will play games with others

Physical examination (particular attention)

Update growth curves.

Continue reassessment; search for new findings.

Examine mouth, and count number of teeth.

Anticipatory guidance

Independence (limit setting, temper tantrums)

Peer interaction

Safety (poisons and potential poisons, water temperature, car safety seat use)

Toilet training

Nightmares

Use of a cup for drinking (as much as possible)

Plans and problems

Review immunizations and implement as appropriate.

Consider need for serum lead level, hemoglobin or hematocrit value, dental referral, tuberculosis test.

Maintain problem list, making appropriate plans and, if necessary, referrals.

3 Years of Age

History (interim details)

Assess parental concerns.
Reassess social and system review.

Development: By this age

Gross motor:
75% will balance on one foot for at least 1 second
75% will negotiate a successful broad jump
40% will balance on one foot for as many as 5 seconds
Fine motor:
80% will copy a circle in addition to a vertical line
80% will build a tower of as many as eight cubes
Language:
Speech is becoming more clearly understood in more than half
80% will use plurals appropriately
Almost half will give their first and last names appropriately
Psychosocial:
90% will put on clothing alone
75% will play interactive games
50% will separate from mother or other significant person
without too much stress
Many will have begun to wash and dry hands

Physical examination (particular attention)

Update growth curves.
Continue reassessment; search for new findings.
Assess whether teeth are coming in appropriately.

Anticipatory guidance

Degrees of independence (limit setting and encouragement, a fine
balance), other aspects of discipline
Safety (car seat, guns, strangers)
Personal hygiene (hand washing, toothbrushing, proper use of
toilet tissue)
Day care

Plans and problems

Review immunizations and implement as appropriate.
Consider need for serum lead level, hemoglobin or hematocrit
value, tuberculosis test.

Maintain problem list, making appropriate plans and, if necessary, referrals.

4 Years of Age

History (interim details)

Assess parental concerns.
Reassess social and system review.

Development: By this age

Gross motor:
75% will hop on one foot
75% will balance on one foot for as many as 5 seconds
65% will be able to imitate a heel-toe walk
Many will have begun to throw overhand
Fine motor:
Almost all will copy a circle and a plus sign
80% will pick longer line of two
50% will begin to draw a person in three parts
Language:
Speech is quite understandable in almost all
95% will give their first and last names
85% will understand *cold, tired, hungry*
80% will identify three of four colors
Psychosocial:
Almost all will play games with other children
70% will dress without supervision

Physical examination (particular attention)

Update growth curves.
Continue reassessment; search for new findings.
Remind that hearing and vision must be evaluated at each visit.
Remind that taking blood pressure is an integral part of physical examination.

Anticipatory guidance

Importance of reading to child frequently
Need for a toddler car seat
Fears and fantasies
Separation (reliance on other adults as time goes by)
Safety (matches and lighters out of reach, strangers, street, window guards)
Personal hygiene (again, importance of frequent toothbrushing)

Plans and problems

Review immunizations, and implement as appropriate.

Consider need for serum lead level, hemoglobin or hematocrit value, urinalysis.

Maintain problem list, making appropriate plans, and if necessary, referrals.

5 Years of Age

History (interim details)

Assess parental concerns.

Reassess social and system review.

Development: By this age

Gross motor:
Almost all will hop nicely on one foot
75% will balance on one foot for as many as 10 seconds
60% will do a heel-toe walk backward reasonably well
Fine motor:
85% will draw a person in three parts
65% will draw a person in as many as six parts
60% will copy a square
Language:
Almost all will identify four colors
Almost all will understand *on, under, in front of, behind*
Well over half will define adequately five of the following eight
words—*ball, cake, desk, house, banana, curtain, fence, ceiling*
Psychosocial:
Almost all will dress without supervision
Almost all will brush teeth without help
Almost all will play board and card games
Almost all will be relaxed when left with a babysitter
More than half will prepare their own cereal

Physical examination (particular attention)

Update growth curves.
Continue reassessment; search for new findings.

Anticipatory guidance

Reading together
School readiness (plays with others, endures separation from parents)

Chores
Discipline (consistency, praising)
Sex identification, education
Peer interaction
Television
Safety (seat belts, guns, bike helmets, matches, swimming; memorize name, address, phone number)

(It is not usually possible to cover so many topics at one visit, so it is usually necessary to be selective based on your knowledge of the family situation.)

Plans and problems

Review immunizations and implement as appropriate.
Consider need for a tuberculosis test, urinalysis.
Maintain problem list, making appropriate plans and, if necessary, referrals.

Elementary School Years (6 to 12 Years of Age)

History (interim details)

Parental concerns
Child's concerns
Reassess social and system review
  Attention span
  Behavior at home and in school
  School accomplishments and experience
  Enuresis, encopresis, constipation, nightmares

Development

By this time gross and fine motor problems have most often become apparent (but not always; neurologic examination should not be shortchanged). Language and psychosocial skills can be readily investigated in talks with parents and child and in explorations of school and play experiences. Socialization and developing maturity may have different expressions at home, on the playground, and in school, and in the variety of times with people of different ages and different degrees of acquaintance. Talks with teachers, report cards, and various drawings and other efforts that the child brings home from school can be very helpful.

Physical examination (particular attention)

Update growth curves.
Continue reassessment; search for new findings.
Begin Tanner stage assessment.

Anticipatory guidance

Parent-child rapport
Need for praise
Responsibility
Safety (seat belts, guns, fire, bike helmets, swimming; memorize
    name, address, phone number)
Allowance
Television
Sex education
Dental care
Adult supervision
Discipline (limit setting)
    *(Again, time constraints almost always make it necessary to adjust
the menu for anticipatory guidance to your judgment about the family's
needs.)*

Plans and problems

Review immunizations and implement as appropriate.
Consider need for a tuberculosis test, urinalysis.
Maintain problem list, making appropriate plans and, if neces-
    sary, referrals.

Adolescents

*(Remember that we have assumed a continuing relationship with the
patient from birth on; real life does not always allow that. If you are see-
ing a patient for the first time, you must, of course, begin with a full history and physical examination.)*

History (interim details)

Patient's concerns
Parental concerns
Menstrual history
Use of tobacco, alcohol, street or other drugs
Diet and what guides it
Sexual activity (relationships, masturbation, pregnancy and dis-
    ease control measures); exact timing for all of this should rely
    on your assessment of the situation and your judgment; in
    general, social experience
School experience
Suicidal ideation; be ever on the alert, and bring it up when nec-
    essary

Update knowledge of home and social structure

Revisit in general social and system review

(An adolescent patient [and some elementary school children] may prefer to be or should be seen alone at times and, as they get older, most often or always. This does not mean, however, that the parents are not involved. Proper balance in this relies on your judgment.)

Development

By this time adolescent's physical, neurologic, and cognitive abilities should be well understood, but nothing should be taken for granted. Conversation with patient, parent or parents, and school officials; school records; and, of course, a careful physical examination should all be helpful.

Physical examination (particular attention)

Update growth curves.

Continue reassessment; search for new findings.

Do Tanner stage assessment.

Assess spinal curvatures, particularly in early adolescent females.

Anticipatory guidance

Puberty and its issues; body image

Sexuality, sexually transmitted disease, contraception

Diet

Tobacco, alcohol, drugs

Risk-taking behavior

Exercise

Safety (guns, seat belts, bike helmets)

Family and other social relationships

Independence and responsibility

School and the future

(Time constraints almost always make it necessary to adjust the menu for anticipatory guidance to your judgment about the adolescent's and/or the family's needs.)

Plans and problems

Review immunizations and implement as appropriate.

Consider need for tuberculosis test, sexually transmitted disease testing, hemoglobin or hematocrit determination, urinalysis, lipid screen.

Maintain problem list, making appropriate plans and, if necessary, referrals.

SPECIAL CONSIDERATIONS FOR THE PREGNANT WOMAN

Use same process of physical examination as for adult.

In addition, perform more extensive abdominal and pelvic evaluations for pregnancy status and fetal well-being.

Late in pregnancy, a woman may find it difficult to assume supine position without experiencing hypotension; use this position only when necessary.

Provide alternative positioning by elevating backrest or by supplying pillows for woman to assume left side-lying position.

Have her empty her bladder to make abdominal assessment more comfortable for her and more accurate.

Remember that during pregnancy, urinary urgency and frequency are common.

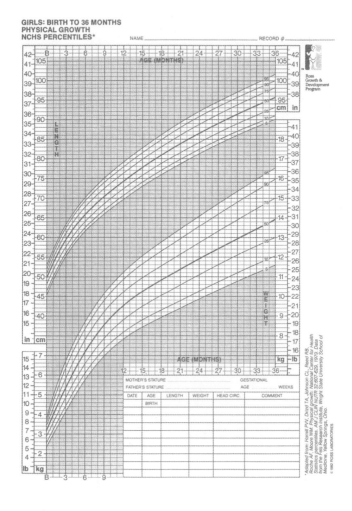

GIRLS: BIRTH TO 36 MONTHS
PHYSICAL GROWTH
NCHS PERCENTILES*

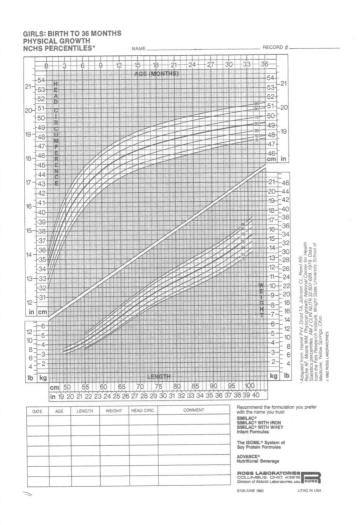

GIRLS: BIRTH TO 36 MONTHS
PHYSICAL GROWTH
NCHS PERCENTILES*

NAME _____ RECORD # _____

BOYS: BIRTH TO 36 MONTHS
PHYSICAL GROWTH
NCHS PERCENTILES*

NAME_____ RECORD #_____

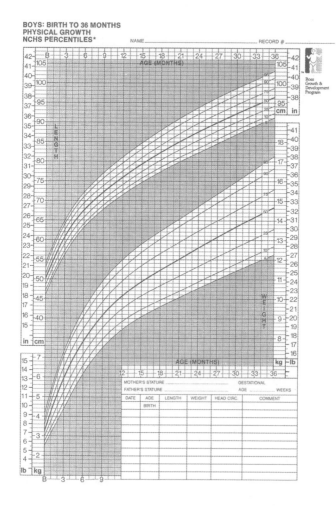

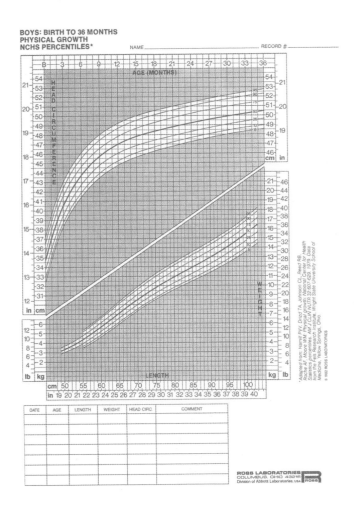

BOYS: BIRTH TO 36 MONTHS
PHYSICAL GROWTH
NCHS PERCENTILES*

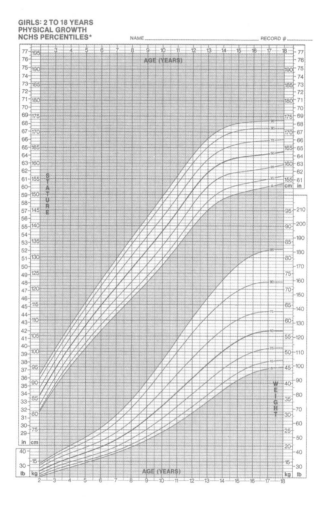

GIRLS: 2 TO 18 YEARS
PHYSICAL GROWTH
NCHS PERCENTILES*

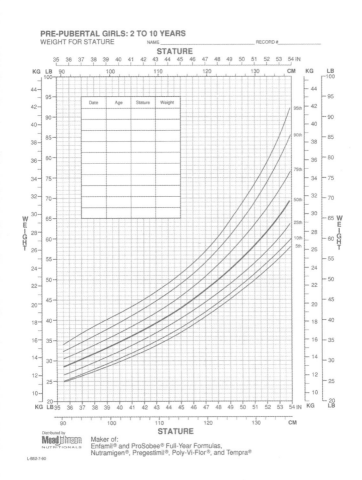

PRE-PUBERTAL GIRLS: 2 TO 10 YEARS
WEIGHT FOR STATURE

Distributed by
Mead Johnson
NUTRITIONALS

Maker of:
Enfamil® and ProSobee® Full-Year Formulas,
Nutramigen®, Pregestimil®, Poly-Vi-Flor®, and Tempra®

L-B52-7-90

BOYS: 2 TO 18 YEARS
PHYSICAL GROWTH
NCHS PERCENTILES*

NAME _____   RECORD # _____

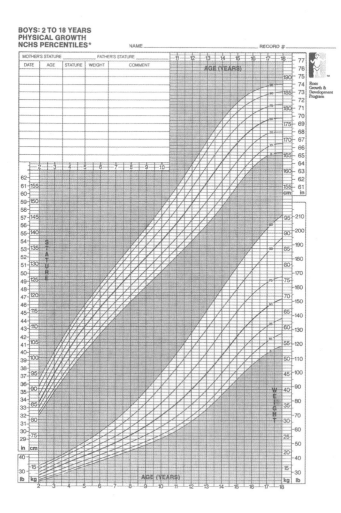

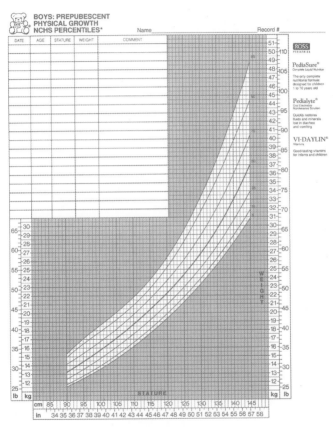

BOYS: PREPUBESCENT
PHYSICAL GROWTH
NCHS PERCENTILES*

Name_____ Record #_____

51212 098W2WB
(0.05)/JUNE 1994

ROSS ROSS PRODUCTS DIVISION
ABBOTT LABORATORIES
COLUMBUS, OHIO 43215-1724

LITHO IN USA

Clinical and Reference Notes

Reporting and Recording

SUBJECTIVE DATA—THE HISTORY

Record the patient's history, especially during an initial visit, to provide a comprehensive database. Arrange information appropriately in specific categories, usually in a particular sequence such as chronologic order with most recent information first. Include both positive and negative data that contribute to the assessment. Use the following organized sequence as a guide.

Identifying Information

Record data recommended by health agency.
  Patient's name
  Identification number/social security number
  Age, sex
  Marital status
  Address (home and business)
  Phone numbers
  Occupation, employer
  Insurance plan, number
  Date of visit
  For children and dependent adults, names of parents or next of
    kin
Put identifying information on each page of record.

Source and Reliability of Information

  Document who is giving the history and relationship to patient.
  Indicate when an old record is used.
  State judgment about reliability of information.

Chief Complaint

Description of patient's main reasons for seeking health care, in patient's own words with quotation marks. Paraphrase only if this makes complaint more clear.

Include duration of problem.

History of Present Problem

List and describe current symptoms of chief complaint and their appearance chronologically in reverse order, dating events and symptoms.

List any expected symptoms that are absent.

Identify anyone in household with same symptoms.

Note pertinent information from review of systems, family history, and personal/social history along with findings.

Where more than one problem is identified, address each in a separate paragraph, including the following details of symptom occurrence:

Onset: When problem first started, chronologic order of events, setting and circumstances, manner of onset (sudden versus gradual)

Location: Exact location, localized or generalized, radiation patterns

Duration: How long problem has lasted, intermittent or continuous, duration of each episode

Character: Nature of symptom

Aggravating/associated factors: Food, activity, rest, certain movements; nausea, vomiting, diarrhea, fever, chills, etc.

Relieving factors: Prescribed and/or self-remedies, alternative or complementary therapies, their effect on the problem; food, rest, heat, ice, activity, position, etc.

Temporal factors: Frequency; relation to other symptoms, problems, functions; symptom improvement or worsening over time

Severity of symptoms: Quantify on a 0 to 10 scale; effect on patient's lifestyle

Medical History

List and describe each of the following with dates of occurrence and any specific information available:

General health and strength over lifetime as patient perceives it; disabilities and functional limitations

Hospitalization and/or surgery: Dates, hospital, diagnosis, complications

Injuries and disabilities

Major childhood illnesses

Adult illnesses and serious injuries

Immunizations: Polio, diphtheria-pertussis-tetanus, tetanus toxoid, influenza, cholera, typhus, typhoid, meningococcal, pneumococcal, bacille Calmette-Guérin (BCG), last purified protein derivative (PPD) or other skin tests, unusual reaction to immunizations

Medications: Past, current, recent medications (prescribed, nonprescription, home remedies); dosages

Allergies: Drugs, foods, environmental

Transfusions: Reason, date, number of units transfused, reactions

Emotional status: History of mood disorders, psychiatric attention or medications

Recent laboratory tests (e.g., cholesterol, Pap smear, mammogram, prostate-specific antigen)

Family history

Present information about age and health of family members in narrative or genogram form, including at least three generations.

Family members: Include parents, grandparents, aunts and uncles, siblings, spouse, children. For deceased family members, note age at time of death and cause, if known.

Major health or genetic disorders: Include hypertension; cancer; cardiac, respiratory, kidney, or thyroid disorders; strokes; asthma or other allergic manifestations; blood dyscrasia; psychiatric difficulties; tuberculosis; diabetes mellitus; hepatitis; or other familial disorders.

Personal/Social History

Include information according to concerns of patient and influence of health problem on patient's and family's life:

Cultural background and practices, birthplace, position in family

Marital status

Religious preference, religious or cultural proscriptions for medical care

Home conditions: Economic condition, number in household, pets

Occupation: Work conditions and hours, physical or mental strain, protective devices used; exposure to chemicals, toxins, poisons, fumes, smoke, asbestos, or radioactive material at home or work

Environment: Home, school, work; structural barriers if handicapped, community services utilized; travel; exposure to contagious diseases

Current health habits and/or risk factors: Exercise; smoking; salt intake; weight control; diet, vitamins and other supplements; caffeine-containing beverages; alcohol or recreational drug use; response to CAGE or TACE questions (see Appendix) related to alcohol use; participation in a drug or alcohol treatment program or support group

Sexual activity: Protection method, contraception

General life satisfaction, hobbies, interests, sources of stress

Review of Systems

Organize in general head-to-toe sequence, including an impression of each symptom.

Record expected or negative findings as absence of symptoms or problems.

When unexpected or positive findings are stated by patient, include details from further inquiry as you would in the present illness.

Include the following categories of information (sequence may vary):

General constitutional symptoms

Diet

Skin, hair, nails

Head and neck

Eyes, ears, nose, mouth, throat

Endocrine

Breasts

Heart and blood vessels

Chest and lungs

Hematologic

Lymphatic, immunologic

Gastrointestinal

Genitourinary

Musculoskeletal

Neurologic

Psychiatric

PHYSICAL FINDINGS
General Statement

Age, race, sex, general appearance
Nutritional status, weight, height, frame size, body mass index
Vital signs: Temperature, pulse rate, respiratory rate, blood pressure (two extremities, two positions)

Mental Status

Physical appearance and behavior
Memory, reasoning, attention span, response to questions
Voice quality, articulation, content, coherence, comprehension
Anxiety, disturbance in thought content

Skin

Color, integrity, temperature, hydration, tattoos
Presence of edema, excessive perspiration, unusual odor
Presence and description of lesions (size, shape, location, inflammation, tenderness, induration, discharge), parasites
Hair texture and distribution
Nail configuration, color, texture, condition, presence of clubbing, nail plate adherence, firmness

Head

Size and contour of head, scalp appearance and movement
Facial features (characteristics, symmetry)
Presence of edema or puffiness, tenderness
Temporal arteries: Characteristics

Eyes

Visual acuity, visual fields
Appearance of orbits, conjunctivae, sclerae, eyelids, eyebrows
Pupillary shape, consensual response to light and accommodation, extraocular movements, corneal light reflex, cover-uncover test
Ophthalmoscopic findings of cornea, lens, retina, optic disc, macula, retinal vessel size, caliber and arteriovenous crossings

Ears

Configuration, position and alignment of auricles
Otoscopic findings of canals (cerumen, lesions, discharge, foreign body) and tympanic membranes (integrity, color, landmarks, mobility, perforation)
Hearing: Air and bone conduction tests, whispered voice

Nose

Appearance of external nose, nasal patency, flaring
Nasal mucosa and septum, color, alignment, discharge, crusting, polyp
Appearance of turbinates
Presence of sinus tenderness or swelling
Discrimination of odors

Mouth and Throat

Number, occlusion and condition of teeth; presence of dental appliances
Lips, tongue, buccal and oral mucosa, floor of mouth (color, moisture, surface characteristics, ulcerations, induration, symmetry)
Oropharynx, tonsils, palate (color, symmetry, exudate)
Symmetry and movement of tongue, soft palate and uvula; gag reflex
Discrimination of taste

Neck

Mobility, suppleness, strength
Position of trachea
Thyroid size, shape, tenderness, nodules
Presence of masses, webbing, skinfolds

Chest

Size and shape of chest, anteroposterior versus transverse diameter, symmetry of movement with respiration
Presence of retractions, use of accessory muscles

Lungs

Respiratory rate, depth, regularity, quietness or ease of respiration
Palpation findings: Symmetry and quality of tactile fremitus, thoracic expansion
Percussion findings: Quality and symmetry of percussion notes, diaphragmatic excursion
Auscultation findings: Characteristics of breath sounds (pitch, duration, intensity, vesicular, bronchial, bronchovesicular) unexpected breath sounds
Characteristics of cough
Presence of friction rub, egophony, whispered pectoriloquy or bronchophony

Breasts

Size, contour

Symmetry, texture, masses, scars, tenderness, thickening, nodules, discharge, retraction, or dimpling

Characteristics of nipples and areolae

Heart

Anatomic location of apical impulse

Heart rate, rhythm, amplitude, contour, symmetry of apical impulse

Palpation findings: Pulsations, thrills, heaves, or lifts

Auscultation findings: Characteristics of S_1 and S_2 (location, intensity, pitch, timing, splitting, systole, diastole)

Presence of murmurs, clicks, snaps, S_3 or S_4 (timing, location, radiation intensity, pitch, quality)

Blood Vessels

Blood pressure: Comparison between extremities, with position change

Jugular vein pulsations and distention, pressure measurement

Presence of bruits over carotid, temporal, renal, and femoral arteries, abdominal aorta

Pulses in distal extremities

Temperature, color, hair distribution, skin texture, nail beds of lower extremities

Presence of edema, swelling, vein distention, Homan sign, or tenderness of lower extremities

Abdomen

Shape, contour, visible aorta pulsations, venous patterns, hernia

Auscultation findings: Bowel sounds in all quadrants, their character

Palpation findings: Aorta, organs, feces, masses, location, size, contour, consistency, tenderness, muscle resistance

Percussion findings: Areas of different percussion notes, costovertebral angle tenderness

Liver span

Male Genitalia

Appearance of external genitalia, circumcision status, location and size of urethral opening, smegma, discharge, lesions, distribution of pubic hair

Palpation findings: Penis, testes, epididymides, vas deferens, contour, consistency, tenderness

Presence of hernia or scrotal swelling

Female Genitalia

Appearance of external genitalia and perineum, distribution of pubic hair, inflammation, excoriation, tenderness, scarring, discharge

Internal examination findings: Appearance of vaginal mucosa, cervix, discharge, odor, lesions

Bimanual examination findings: Size, position, tenderness of cervix, vaginal walls, uterus, adnexa, ovaries

Rectovaginal examination findings

Urinary incontinence with bearing down

Anus and Rectum

Sphincter control, presence of hemorrhoids, fissures, skin tags, polyps

Rectal wall contour, tenderness, sphincter tone

Prostate size, contour, consistency, mobility

Color and consistency of stool

Lymphatic

Presence of lymph nodes in head, neck, epitrochlear, axillary, or inguinal areas

Size, shape, consistency, warmth, tenderness, mobility, discreteness of nodes

Musculoskeletal

Posture: Alignment of extremities and spine, symmetry of body parts

Symmetry of muscle mass, tone and strength; grading of strength, fasciculations, spasms

Range of motion, passive and active; presence of pain with movement

Appearance of joints; presence of deformities, tenderness or crepitus

Neurologic

Cranial nerves: Specific findings for each or specify those tested, if findings are recorded in head and neck sections

Cerebellar and motor function: Gait, balance, coordination with
rapid alternating motions

Sensory function, symmetry (touch, pain, vibration, temperature,
monofilament)

Superficial and deep tendon reflexes: Symmetry, grade

ASSESSMENT

Diagnoses with rationale, based on subjective and objective data
Anticipated potential problems
Disease progression or complication
New problem

PLAN

Diagnostic tests ordered or performed
Therapeutic treatment plan
Patient education
Referrals initiated
Future visit to evaluate plan

Clinical and Reference Notes

Appendix

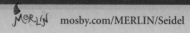

Quick Reference to Special Histories

CAGE Questionnaire: A Framework for Detecting Alcoholism

Mnemonic	Questions
C: Concern, cut down	Have you ever been concerned about your own or someone else's drinking? Have you ever felt the need to cut down on drinking? Probe: What was it like? Were you successful? Why did you decide to cut down?
A: Annoyed	Have you ever felt annoyed by criticism of your drinking? Probe: What caused the worry or concern? Do you ever get irritated by others' worries? Have you ever limited what you drink to please someone?
G: Guilty	Have you ever felt guilty about your drinking? Have you ever felt guilty about something you said or did while you were drinking? Probe: Have you ever been bothered by anything you have done or said while you've been drinking? Have you ever regretted anything that has happened to you while you were drinking?
E: Eye-opener	Have you ever felt the need for a morning eye-opener drink? Probe: Have you ever felt shaky or tremulous after a night of heavy drinking? What did you do to relieve the shakiness? Have you ever had trouble getting back to sleep early in the morning after a night of heavy drinking?

From Ewing, 1998.

TACE Questionnaire: A Framework for Prenatal Detection of Risk Drinking

Mnemonic	Questions
T: Take	How many drinks does it take to make you feel high? (More than two drinks suggests a tolerance to alcohol that is a red flag.) How many when you first started drinking? When was that? Which do you prefer: beer, wine, or liquor?
A: Annoyed	Have people annoyed you by criticizing your drinking?
C: Cut down	Have you felt you ought to cut down on your drinking?
E: Eye-opener	Have you ever had an eye-opener drink first thing in the morning to steady your nerves or get rid of a hangover?

A positive answer to T alone or to two of A, C, or E may signal a problem with a high degree of probability, and positive answers to all four, with great certainty.

From Sokol, Martier, Ager, 1989.

The RAFFT Questionnaire: A Framework for Detecting Substance Use Disorders in Adolescents

Mnemonic	Questions
T: Take	How many drinks does it take to make you feel high? (More than two drinks suggests a tolerance to alcohol that is a red flag.) How many when you first started drinking? When was that? Which do you prefer: beer, wine, or liquor?
R: Relax	Do you drink or take drugs to relax, feel better about yourself, or fit in?
A: Alone	Do you ever drink or take drugs while you are alone?
F: Friends	Do any of your closest friends drink or use drugs?
F: Family	Does a close family member have a problem with alcohol or drugs?
T: Trouble	Have you ever gotten into trouble from drinking or taking drugs?

From Bastiaens, Francis, Lewis, 2000.

Domestic Violence: Three Questions as a Brief Screening Instrument

1. Have you been hit, kicked, punched, or otherwise hurt by someone within the past year?
2. Do you feel safe in your current relationship?
3. Is a partner from a previous relationship making you feel un-safe now?

A positive response to any one of the three questions constitutes a positive screen for partner violence.

The first question, which addresses physical violence, has been validated in studies as an accurate measure of 1-year prevalence rates.

The last two questions evaluate the perception of safety and esti-mate the short-term risk of further violence and the need for counseling, but reliability and validity evaluations have not yet been established

From Feldhaus et al, 1997.

BATHE Questionnaire: A Framework for Understanding the Patient in the Context of His or Her Total Life Situation

Mnemonic	Questions
B: Background	What is going on in your life?
	What is going on right now?
	Has anything changed recently?
A: Affect	How do you feel about that?
	What is your mood?
T: Trouble	What about the situation troubles you most?
	What worries or concerns you?
H: Handling	How are you handling that?
	How are you coping?
E: Empathy	That must be very difficult for you.
	I can understand that you would feel that way.

From Stuart, Lieberman, 1993; and Lieberman, 1997.

HOPE Questionnaire: A Framework for Spiritual Assessment

Mnemonic	Questions
H: Hope—sources of hope, meaning, comfort, strength, peace, love, and connection	We have been discussing your support systems. I was wondering, what is there in your life that gives you internal support? What are your sources of hope, strength, comfort, and peace? What do you hold on to during difficult times? What sustains you and keeps you going? For some people, their religious or spiritual beliefs act as a source of comfort and strength in dealing with life's ups and downs; is this true for you? If the answer is yes, go on to O and P questions. If the answer is no, consider asking, "Was it ever?" If the answer is yes, ask, "What changed?"
O: Organized religion	Do you consider yourself part of an organized religion? How important is this to you? What aspects of your religion are helpful and not so helpful to you? Are you part of a religious or spiritual community? Does is help you? How?
P: Personal spirituality/practices	Do you have personal spiritual beliefs that are independent of organized religion? What are they? Do you believe in God? What kind of relationship do you have with God?

	What aspects of your spirituality or spiritual practices do you find most helpful to you personally? (Examples include prayer, meditation, reading scripture, attending religious services, listening to music, hiking, communing with nature.)
E: Effects on medical care and end-of-life issues	Has being sick (or your current situation) affected your ability to do the things that usually help you spiritually (or affected your relationship with God)?
	As a doctor, is there anything that I can do to help you access the resources that usually help you?
	Are you worried about any conflicts between your beliefs and your medical situation/care/decisions?
	Would it be helpful for you to speak to a clinical chaplain/community spiritual leader?
	Are there any specific practices or restrictions I should know about in providing your medical care (e.g., dietary restrictions, use of blood products)?
	If the patient is dying: How do your beliefs affect the kind of medical care you would like me to provide over the next few days/weeks/months?

Anandarajah, Hight, 2001.

SPIRIT Questionnaire: A Framework for Spiritual Assessment

Mnemonic	Questions
S: Spiritual belief system	What is your formal religious affiliation? Name or describe your spiritual belief system.
P: Personal spirituality	Describe the beliefs and practices of your religion or spiritual system that you personally accept. Describe the beliefs or practices you do not accept. Do you accept or believe (specific tenet or practice)? What does your spirituality/religion mean to you? What is the importance of your spirituality/religion in daily life?
I: Integration with a spiritual community	Do you belong to any spiritual or religious group or community? What is your position or role? What importance does this group have to you? Is it a source of support? In what ways? Does or could this group provide help in dealing with health issues?

R: Ritualized practices and restrictions	Are there specific practices that you carry out as part of your religion/spirituality (e.g., prayer or meditation)?
	Are there certain lifestyle activities or practices that your religion/spirituality encourages or forbids? Do you comply? What significance do these practices and restrictions have to you?
	Are there specific elements of medical care that you forbid on the basis of religious/spiritual grounds?
I: Implications for medical care	What aspects of your religion/spirituality would you like me to keep in mind as I care for you?
	Would you like to discuss religious or spiritual implications of health care?
	What knowledge or understanding would strengthen our relationship as physician and patient?
	Are there any barriers to our relationship based on religious or spiritual issues?
T: Terminal events planning	As we plan for your care near the end of life, how does your faith affect your decisions?
	Are there particular aspects of care that you wish to forgo or have withheld because of your faith?

From Maugans, 1996.

ETHNIC Questionnaire: A Framework for Culturally Competent Clinical Practice

Mnemonic	Questions
E: Explanation	Why do you think you have these symptoms? What do friends, family, and others say? Do you know others with this problem? Have you seen it on TV, heard about it on the radio, or read about it in the newspaper?
T: Treatment	Do you take any treatments, medicines, or home remedies to treat the illness or to stay healthy? What kinds of treatment are you seeking from me?
H: Healers	Have you sought advice from friends, alternative folk healers, or other nondoctors?
N: Negotiate	Negotiate mutually acceptable options; incorporate patient's beliefs. Ask results patient hopes to achieve from intervention.
I: Intervention	Determine an intervention with your patient. May include incorporation of alternative treatments, spirituality, healers, or other cultural practices (e.g., foods to be eaten or avoided).
C: Collaborate	Collaborate with the patient, family, health team members, healers, and community resources.

Modified from Levin et al, 1997.

References

Adams JA: Evolution of a classification scale: medical evaluation of suspected child sexual abuse, *Child Maltreat* 6:31-36, 2001.

Agency for Healthcare Research and Quality: *Management of acute otitis media: Summary, evidence report/technology assessment No. 15,* Rockville, Md, June 2000, The Agency; http://www.ahrq.gov/clinic/otitisum.htm.

Ahuja V, Yencha MW, Lassen LF: Head and neck manifestations of gastro-esophageal reflux disease, *Am Fam Physician* 50(3):873-880, 885-886, 1999.

American Academy of Pediatrics: Guidelines for the evaluation of sexual abuse of children: subject review (RE 9819), *Pediatrics* 103(1):186-191, 1999.

American Academy of Pediatrics: *Policy statement RE 9850,* Elk Grove Village, Ill, March 1999, The Academy.

American Academy of Pediatrics Committee on Quality Improvement, Subcommittee on Developmental Dysphasia of the Hip: Clinical practice guideline: early detection of developmental dysphasia of the hip, *Pediatrics* 105(4):896-905, 2000.

American Academy of Pediatrics Committee on Sports Medicine and Fitness: Medical conditions affecting sports participation, *Pediatrics* 107(5):1205-1209, 2001.

American Cancer Society: http://www.cancer.org/, accessed 2000.

Anandarajah G, Hight E: Spirituality and medical practice: using the HOPE questions as a practical tool for spiritual assessment, *Am Fam Physician* 63(1):81-89, 2001.

Apantaku LM: Breast cancer diagnosis and screening, *Am Fam Physician* 62(3):596-602, 2000.

Arvidson CR: The adolescent gynecologic exam, *Pediatr Nurs* 25(1):71-74, 1999.

Athey J, Moody-Williams J: *Serving disaster survivors: achieving cultural competence in crisis counseling,* Washington, DC, 2000, Emergency Services and Disaster Relief Branch, Center for Mental Health Services, Substance Abuse and Mental Health Services Administration.

Attia MW et al: Performance of a predictive model for streptococcal pharyngitis in children, *Arch Pediatr Adolesc Med* 155:687-691, 2001.

Bacal DA, Wilson MC: Strabismus: getting it straight, *Contemp Pediatr* 17:49, 2000.

Baran R, Dawber RPR, Levene G: *Color atlas of the hair, scalp and nails,* St Louis, 1991, Mosby.

Barkauskas VH et al: *Health and physical assessment,* ed 3, St Louis, 2001, Mosby.

Bastiaens L, Francis G, Lewis K: The RAFFT as a screening tool for adolescent substance use disorders, *Am J Addict* 9(1):10-16, 2000.

Bluestone CD, Klein JO: *Otitis media in infants and children,* ed 3, Philadelphia, 2001, WB Saunders.

Brooke P, Bullock R: Validation of a 6-item cognitive impairment test with a view to primary care, *Int J Geriatr Psychiatry* 14(1):936-940, 1999.

Brown JE, Carlson M: Nutrition and multi-fetal pregnancy, *J Am Diet Assoc* 100(3):343-348, 2000.

Burrow GN: Thyroid diseases. In Burrow GN, Duffy TP, editors: *Medical complications during pregnancy,* ed 5. Philadelphia, 1999, WB Saunders.

Castiglia PT: Depression in children, *J Pediatr Health Care* 14(2):73-75, 2000.

Caulin-Glaser T, Setaro J: Pregnancy and cardiovascular disease. In Burrow GN, Duffy TP, editors: *Medical complications during pregnancy,* ed 5, Philadelphia, 1999, WB Saunders.

Centers for Disease Control and Prevention: *Standard precautions,* http://www.cdc./gov/ncidod/hip/guide/guide.htm, updated May 15, 2000.

Centers for Disease Control and Prevention: http://www.cdc.gov/ncidod/diseases/hepatitis/index.htm, revised October 20, 2000.

Christensen FC, Rayburn WF: Fetal movement counts, *Obstet Gynecol Clin North Am* 26(4):607-621, 1999.

Clark D: Immunology of pregnancy. In Burrow GN, Duffy TP, editors: *Medical complications of pregnancy,* ed 5, Philadelphia, 1999, WB Saunders.

D'Arcy CA, McGee S: Does this patient have carpal tunnel syndrome? *JAMA* 283(23):3110-3117, 2000.

Deering CG: To speak or not to speak: self-closure with patients, *AJN Am J Neuroradiol* 99:34-38, 1999.

Delves PJ, Roitt IM: The immune system, *N Engl J Med* 343:108-116, 2000.

Donaldson JO: Neurologic complications. In Burrow GN, Duffy TP, editors: *Medical complications during pregnancy,* ed 5, Philadelphia, 1999, WB Saunders.

Dowd Ravalieri RJ: Help your patient live with osteoporosis, *AJN Am J Neuroradiol* 99(4):55-60, 1999.

Edge V, Miller M: *Women's health care,* St Louis, 1994, Mosby.

Ewing JA: Screening for alcoholism using CAGE: cut down, annoyed, guilty, eye opener, *JAMA* 280(2):1904-1905, 1998.

Executive Summary of the Third Report of the National Cholesterol Education Program Expert Panel on Detection, Evaluation, and Treatment of High Blood Cholesterol in Adults (Adult Treatment Panel III), *JAMA* 285(19):2486-2497, 2001.

Farrar WE, et al: *Infectious diseases,* ed 2, London, 1992, Gower.

Feldhaus K, et al: Accuracy of 3 brief screening questions for detecting partner violence in the emergency department, *JAMA* 277(17):1357-1361, 1997.

Ferrie B: Complementary modalities in the new millennium, *Advance for Nursing* May 3:28-29, 1999.

Folstein M et al: The meaning of cognitive impairment in the elderly, *J Am Geriatr Soc* 33(4):228, 1985.

Folstein MF et al: "Mini-Mental State": a practical method for grading the cognitive state of patients for the clinician, *J Psychiatr Res* 12:189, 1975.

Franklin SS et al: Is pulse pressure useful in prediction risk for coronary heart disease? *Circulation* 100:354, 1999.

Frisancho AR: New norms of upper limb fat and muscle areas for assessment of nutritional status, *Am J Clin Nutr* 34:2540, 1981.

Frisancho AR: New standards of weight and body composition by frame size and height for assessment of nutritional status of adults and the elderly, *Am J Clin Nutr* 40:808, 1984.

Gardosi J, Francis A: Controlled trial of fundal height measurement plotted on customized antenatal growth charts, *Br J Obstet Gynecol* 104(4):309-317, 1999.

Goldman MP, Fitzpatrick RE: *Cutaneous laser surgery: the art and science of selective photothermolysis,* ed 2, St Louis, 1999, Mosby.

Gotzsche PC, Olsen O: Is screening for breast cancer with mammography justifiable? *Lancet* 355(9198):129-134, 2000.

Habif TP: *Clinical dermatology,* ed 3, St Louis, 1996, Mosby.

Haller CA, Benowitz NL: Adverse cardiovascular and central nervous system events associated with dietary supplements containing ephedra alkaloids, *N Engl J Med* 343:1833-1842, 2000.

Hardie GE et al: Ethnic descriptors used by African-American and white asthma patients during induced bronchoconstriction, *Chest* 117:935-943, 2000.

Harvey AM et al: *The principles and practice of medicine,* ed 22, Norwalk, Conn, 1988, Appleton & Lange.

Hennigan L, Kollar LM, Rosenthal SL: Methods for managing pelvic examination anxiety: individual differences and relaxation techniques, *J Pediatr Health Care* 14(1):9-12, 2000.

Hoberman A, Paradise JL: Acute otitis media: diagnosis and management in the year 2000, *Pediatr Ann* 29(10):609-620, 2000.

Jacobson A: Research for practice: saving limbs with Semmes-Weinstein monofilament, *AJN Am J Neuroradiol* 99(2):76, 1999.

Jacobson RD: Approach to the child with weakness and clumsiness, *Pediatr Clin North Am* 45(1):145-168, 1998.

Jerant AF et al: Early detection and treatment of skin cancer, *Am Fam Physician* 62(2):357-368, 375-376, 381-382, 2000.

Johnson TS et al: Reliability of three length measurement techniques in term infants, *Pediatr Nurs* 25(1):13-17, 1999.

Judge R et al: *Clinical diagnosis,* ed 5, Boston, 1988, Little, Brown.

Kahn JA, Emans SJ: Gynecologic examination of the prepubertal girl, *Contemp Pediatr* 16(3):148-159, 1999.

Kaplowitz PB, Oberfield SE, the Drug and Therapeutics and Executive Committees of the Lawson Wilkins Pediatric Endocrine Society: Reexamination of the age limits for defining when puberty is precocious in girls in the United States: implications for evaluation and treatment, *Pediatrics* 104(4):936-941, 1999.

Kennedy CT, Kyle P: Skin diseases. In James DK et al, editors: *High-risk pregnancy: management options,* ed 2, Philadelphia, 1999, WB Saunders.

Kerker BD et al: Identification of violence in the home, *Arch Pediatr Adolesc Med* 154:457-462, 2000.

Kernan WN et al: Phenylpropanolamine and risk of hemorrhagic stroke, *N Engl J Med* 343:1826-1832, 2000.

Khandker RK et al: A decision model and cost-effectiveness analysis of colorectal cancer screening and surveillance guidelines for average-risk adults, *Int J Technol Assess Health Care* 16(3):799-810, 2000.

Knight JR et al: A new brief screen for adolescent substance abuse, *Arch Pediatr Adolesc Med* 153:591-596, 1999.

Knight JR et al: Reliabilities of short substance abuse screening tests among adolescent medical patients, *Pediatrics* 105:948-953, 2000.

Koop CE: *The Surgeon General's letter on child sexual abuse,* Rockville, Md, 1988, U.S. Department of Health and Human Services.

Kuczmarski MF, Kuczmarski RJ, Najjar M: Descriptive anthropometric reference data for older Americans, *J Am Diet Assoc* 100:59-66, 2000.

Lanham DM et al: Accuracy of tympanic temperature readings in children under 6 years of age, *Pediatr Nurs* 25(1):39-42, 1999.

Lapinsky S: Cardiopulmonary changes in pregnancy: what you need to know, *Women's Health in Primary Care* 2:353, 1999.

Lemmi FO, Lemmi CAE: *Physical assessment findings CD-ROM,* Philadelphia, 2000, WB Saunders.

Levin S, Like R, Gottlieb J, Department of Family Medicine, University of Medicine and Dentistry of New Jersey, Robert Wood Johnson Medical School: *ETHNIC: A framework for culturally competent clinical practice,* 1997.

Lieberman JA III: BATHE: an approach to the interview process in the primary care setting, *J Clin Psychiatry* 58(suppl 3):3-6, 1997.

Lipman TH et al: Assessment of growth by primary health care providers, *J Pediatr Health Care* 14(4):166-171, 2000.

Lowdermilk DL, Perry SE, Bobak IM: *Maternity and women's health care,* ed 7, St Louis, 2000, Mosby.

Mattson JE: The language of pain, *Reflections on Nursing Leadership* Fourth quarter:11-14, 2000.

Maugans TA: The SPIRITual history, *Arch Fam Med* 5(1):11-16, 1996.

McCaffery M, Pasero C: Teaching patients to use a numerical pain-rating scale, *AJN Am J Neuroradiol* 99:22, 1999.

McCarty DJ: *Arthritis and allied conditions: a textbook of rheumatology,* ed 2, Philadelphia, 1993, Lea & Febiger.

McClain N et al: Evaluation of sexual abuse in the pediatric patient, *Pediatric Health Care* 14(3): 93-102, 2000.

McNeese M: Evaluation of sexual abuse in the pediatric patient, *J Pediatr Health Care* 14(3):93-102, 2000.

Mendelson M, Lang R: Pregnancy and cardiovascular disease. In Barron WM, Lindheimer MD, Davison JM, editors: *Medical disorders during pregnancy,* ed 3, St Louis, 2000, Mosby.

Miyasaki-Ching CM: *Chasteen's essentials of clinical dental assisting,* ed 5, St Louis, 1997, Mosby.

Modigliani RM: Gastrointestinal and pancreatic disorders. In Barron WM, Lindheimer MD, Davison JM, editors: *Medical disorders during pregnancy,* ed 3, St Louis, 2000, Mosby.

Molitch M: Pituitary, thyroid, adrenal, and parathyroid disorders. In Barron WM, Lindheimer MD, Davison JM, editors: *Medical disorders during pregnancy,* ed 3, St Louis, 2000, Mosby.

Moody CW: Male child sexual abuse, *J Pediatr Health Care* 13:112-119, 1999.

Morrow M: The evaluation of common breast problems, *Am Fam Physician* 61(8):2371-2378, 2385, 2000.

Moyer LA, Mast EE, Altre MJ: Hepatitis C: Part II. Prevention counseling and medical evaluation, *Am Fam Physician* 59(2):349-354, 357, 1999.

National Cholesterol Education Program Expert Panel on Detection, Evaluation, and Treatment of High Blood Cholesterol in Adults: Executive summary of the third report of the National Cholesterol Education Program (NCEP) Expert Panel on Detection, Evaluation, and Treatment of High Blood Cholesterol (Adult Treatment Panel III), *JAMA* 285(19):2486-2497, 2001.

National Institutes of Health: *Report No. 48-4080,* Bethesda, Md, November 1997, The Institutes.

Naway H et al: Concordance of clinical findings and clinical judgment in diagnosis of streptococcal pharyngitis, *Acad Emerg Med* 7(10):1104-1109, 2000.

Nuss R, Manco-Johnson MJ: Venous thrombosus: issues for the pediatrician, *Contemp Pediatr* 17:75, 2000.

Ramsburg KL: Rheumatoid arthritis, *AJN Am J Neuroradiol* 100(11):40-43, 2000.

Reifsnider E, Gill S: Nutrition for the childbearing years, *J Obstet Gynecol Neonatal Nurs* 29(1):43-45, 2000.

Rex DK et al: Colorectal cancer prevention 2000: screening recommendations of the American College of Gastroenterology, *Am J Gastroenterol* 95:868-877, 2000.

Rose VL: CDC issues new recommendations for the prevention and control of hepatitis C virus infection, *Am Fam Physician* 59(5):1321-1323, 1999.

Rosenthal TC, Puck SM: Screening for genetic risk of breast cancer, *Am Fam Physician* 59(1):99-104, 106, 1999.

Rudy ED: *Advanced neurological and neurosurgical nursing,* St Louis, 1984, Mosby.

Samiy AH, Douglas RG Jr, Barondess JA: *Textbook of diagnostic medicine,* Philadelphia, 1987, Lea & Febiger.

Schairer C et al: Menopausal estrogen and estrogen-progestin replacement therapy and breast cancer risk, *JAMA* 283(4):485-491, 2000.

Schulman KA et al: The effects of race and sex on physician's recommendations for cardiac catheterization, *N Engl J Med* 340:618-626, 1999.

Scott M, Gelhot AR: Gastroesophageal reflux disease: diagnosis and management, *Am Fam Physician* 59(5):1161-1169, 1199, 1999.

Seidel HM, et al: *Mosby's guide to physical examination,* ed 5, St Louis: Mosby, 2003.

Sheikh JL, Yesavage JA: Geriatric depression scale: recent evidence and development of a shorter version, *Clin Gerontol* 5:165-172, 1986.

Shinitzky HE, Kub J: The art of motivating behavior change: the use of motivational interviewing to promote health, *Public Health Nurs* 18:178-185, 2001.

Sloan RP et al: Should physicians prescribe religious activities? *N Engl J Med* 342:1913-1916, 2000.

Smith RD, McNamara JJ: The neurological examination of children with school problems, *J Sch Health* 54(7):231-234, 1984.

Sokol RJ, Martier SS, Ager JW: TACE questions: practical prenatal detection of risk-drinking, *Am J Obstet Gynecol* 260(4):863-868, 1989.

Stang J: Adolescent physical growth and development: implications for pregnancy. In Story M, Stang J, editors: *Nutrition and the pregnant adolescent,* Minneapolis, Minn, 2000, Center for Leadership, Education, and Training in Maternal and Children Nutrition, University of Minnesota.

Star W et al: *Ambulatory obstetrics,* ed 3. San Francisco, 1999, UCSF Nursing Press.

Starr NB, Poland C, Dean JA: Malocclusion: How important is that bite? *J Pediatr Health Care* 13:245-247, 1999.

Stuart MR, Lieberman JA III: *The fifteen minute hour: applied psychotherapy for the primary care physician,* ed 2, New York, 1993, Praeger.

Teoh TG, Fisk NM: Hydramnios, oligohydramnios. In James DK et al, editors: *High risk pregnancy: management options,* ed 2, Philadelphia, 1999, WB Saunders.

Thibodeau GA, Patton KT: *Anatomy & physiology,* ed 4, St Louis, 1999, Mosby.

Thomas AE et al: A nomogram method for assessing body weight, *Am J Clin Nutr* 29(3):302-304, 1976.

Thompson JM, Wilson SF: *Health assessment for nursing practice,* St Louis, 1996, Mosby.

Thompson JM et al: *Mosby's clinical nursing,* ed 4, St Louis, 1997, Mosby.

U.S. Department of Health and Human Services: *Clinician's handbook of preventive services,* Washington, DC, 1994, U.S. Government Printing Office.

U.S. Preventive Services Task Force: *Guide to clinical preventive services,* ed 2, Washington, DC, 1996, U.S. Government Printing Office.

Varcarolis EM: *Psychiatric nursing clinical guide: assessment tools and diagnosis,* Philadelphia, 1999, WB Saunders.

Videlefsky A et al: Routine vaginal cuff smear testing in post-hysterectomy patients with benign uterine conditions: When is it indicated? *J Am Board Fam Pract* 13(4):233-238, 2000.

Warner PH, Rowe T, Whipple B: Shedding light on the sexual history, *AJN Am J Neuroradiol* 99:34-40, 1999.

Weinberger S, Weiss S: Pulmonary diseases. In Burrow GN, Duffy TP, editors: *Medical complications of pregnancy,* ed 5, Philadelphia, 1999, WB Saunders.

Weiner CP, Baschat AA: Fetal growth restriction: evaluation and management. In James DK et al, editors: *High risk pregnancy: management options,* ed 2, Philadelphia, 1999, WB Saunders.

Werk LN, Bauchner H, Chessare JB: Medicine for the millennium: demystifying EBM, *Contemp Pediatr* 16:87-107, 1999.

Weston WL, Lane AT, Mortelli JG: *Color textbook of pediatric dermatology,* ed 2, St Louis, 1996, Mosby.

White GM: *Color atlas of regional dermatology,* St Louis, 1994, Mosby.

Whooley MA, Simon GE: Managing depression in medical outpatients, *N Engl J Med* 343:1942-1950, 2000.

Wilson MEH: Keeping quiet, *Arch Pediatr Adolesc Med* 152:1054-1055, 1999.

Wilson SF, Giddens JF: *Health assessment for nursing practice,* ed 2, St Louis, 2001, Mosby.

Wong DL, et al: *Whaley and Wong's nursing care of infants and children,* ed 6, St Louis, 1999, Mosby.

Wong DL, et al: *Wong's essentials of pediatric nursing,* ed 6, St Louis, 2001, Mosby.

Wright RJ: Identification of violence in the community pediatric setting, *Arch Pediatr Adolesc Med* 154:431-433, 2000.

Zitelli BJ, Davis HW: *Atlas of pediatric physical diagnosis,* ed 3, St Louis, 1997, Mosby.

Zlatnik F et al: Vaginal ultrasound as an adjunct to cervical digital examination in women at risk for early delivery, *Gynecol Obstet Invest* 51(1):12-16, 2001.

Index